# 人体血管铸型及血管造影
# 彩色图谱

主　编　孙国生　李洪鹏　李　波
主　审　隋鸿锦　王兴海

U0323458

辽宁科学技术出版社
·沈阳·

**图书在版编目（CIP）数据**

人体血管铸型及血管造影彩色图谱/孙国生，李洪鹏，李波
主编. —沈阳：辽宁科学技术出版社，2018.4
ISBN 978-7-5591-0609-4

Ⅰ.①人⋯　Ⅱ.①孙⋯　②李⋯　③李⋯　Ⅲ.①血管外科学—
人体解剖学—图谱　②血管造影—图谱　Ⅳ.①R654.3-64
②R816.2-64

中国版本图书馆CIP数据核字（2017）第330024号

出版发行：辽宁科学技术出版社
　　　　　（地址：沈阳市和平区十一纬路25号　邮编：110003）
印　刷　者：辽宁新华印务有限公司
经　销　者：各地新华书店
幅面尺寸：185mm×260mm
印　　张：8.5
字　　数：220千字
出版时间：2018年4月第1版
印刷时间：2018年4月第1次印刷
责任编辑：郭敬斌
封面设计：刘　丰
版式设计：袁　舒
责任校对：李　霞

书　　号：ISBN 978-7-5591-0609-4
定　　价：98.00元

联系电话：024-23284363
邮购热线：024-23284502
邮　　箱：guojingbin@126.com

# 编委会

主　编　孙国生　李洪鹏　李　波
副主编　韩　建　吴松林　王万粮
主　审　隋鸿锦　王兴海
编　委（以姓氏笔画为序）

王　顺　中国医科大学

王万粮　沈阳医学院附属第二医院

东　洋　沈阳医学院附属第二医院

朱　巍　沈阳医学院附属第二医院

刘继辉　中国医科大学附属第一医院

孙永林　大连鸿峰生物科技有限公司

孙国生　沈阳体育学院

孙翔宇　大连鸿峰生物科技有限公司

李　波　中国医科大学附属口腔医院

李洪鹏　中国医科大学

李慧有　大连鸿峰生物科技有限公司

吴　敏　沈阳体育学院

吴松林　沈阳体育学院

佟　瑶　沈阳体育学院

陈　新　沈阳体育学院

林洪春　沈阳体育学院

郑　岩　大连鸿峰生物科技有限公司

高　岩　沈阳体育学院

郭中献　郑州国希望教学用品有限公司

韩　建　大连鸿峰生物科技有限公司

甄希成　沈阳体育学院

**标本制作**　张党谋　李忠华　李泽宇　吴坤成　刘健华　孙翔宇　孙国生　刘　海
**摄影及图片处理**　刘　畅　赵　欣

# 前 言

本图谱遵照《全国高等医学院校解剖教学大纲》的要求，系统展示了人体循环系统的分布及走向。目前国内已有多种人工绘制或实物标本的解剖图谱，这些图谱在我国的解剖教学和临床医疗工作中发挥了重要作用。

随着解剖教学改革的不断深入，教学学时逐渐减少，教学内容不断精简，学生及广大教师、临床医务工作者，在教材中所学到的知识和在实验室看到的标本与教材图谱有很大的不同，特别是进入临床工作以后，更觉得书本上所描述的知识和解剖图谱所显示的内容无法满足工作需要，尤其临床上应用最广泛的人体心血管系统，个体变异显著。在教学、医疗和科研工作中，图像占有非常重要的地位，无论是在基础医学还是临床教学中，除使用文字教材外，还必须提供大量的标本及影像图像，特别是随着科学技术的不断发展与进步，新的医学影像仪器设备的投入，信息技术、3D打印等技术的大量应用，使图像的分辨率提高，图像在疾病诊断中日益成为不可或缺的重要手段之一。

为了给学生、教师及广大临床医务工作者提供比较充分的图像资源，我们编绘了医学教学与应用图谱《人体血管铸型及血管造影彩色图谱》，本图谱分为五部分：头颈部血管、胸腹部血管、盆部血管、上肢血管、下肢血管。在本书编写过程中，参考了柏树令教授等主编的《系统解剖学》第8版，宋国华教授、王兴海教授主编的《全彩人体心血管学图谱》。本图谱所用的标本及病例由南方医科大学、郑州国希望教学用品有限公司、大连鸿峰生物科技有限公司、中国医科大学附属第一医院、沈阳医学院附属第二医院等单位提供。本图谱在编写过程中得到了辽宁科学技术出版社社长宋纯智及责任编辑郭敬斌老师的大力支持，在此对给予帮助的同仁表示衷心感谢。

由于本书的编写时间比较仓促，作者的学术水平和编写能力有限，难免出现内容和文字上的疏漏和错误，恳请学界同仁及临床医务工作者提出批评斧正，使其臻于完善。

孙国生
2016年夏于沈阳体育学院

# 目　录

**胸腹部血管**

## 盆部血管

# 上肢血管

## 下肢血管

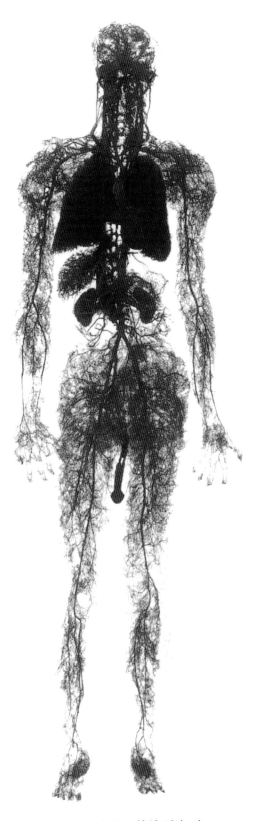

图1-1　全身血管铸型（1）
the cast at every bore（1）

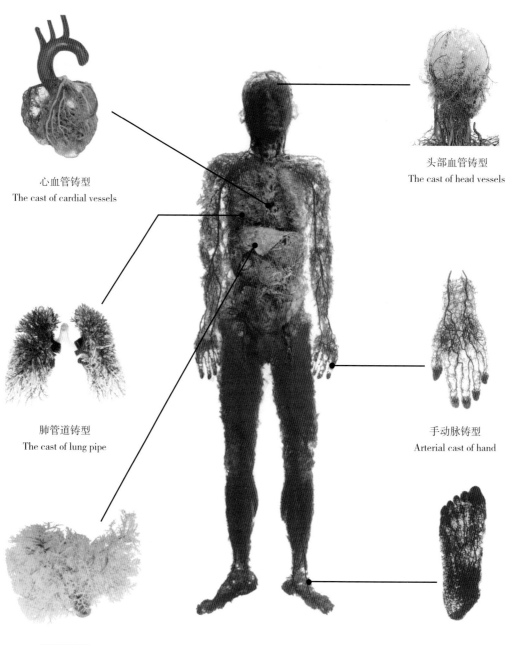

心血管铸型
The cast of cardial vessels

头部血管铸型
The cast of head vessels

肺管道铸型
The cast of lung pipe

手动脉铸型
Arterial cast of hand

肝管道铸型
The cast of hepatic duct

足动脉铸型
Arterial cast of foot

图1-2　全身血管铸型（2）
the cast at every bore（2）

# 头颈部血管

孙国生　孙翔宇　李洪鹏

李　波　陈　新　刘继辉

1. 颞浅动脉额支 frontal branch of superficial temporal artery
2. 眶上动脉 supraorbital artery
3. 泪腺动脉 lacrimal artery
4. 颞深动脉 deep temporal artery
5. 耳动脉 auricular artery
6. 眶下动脉 infraorbital artery
7. 内眦动脉 angular artery
8. 眼动脉 ophthalmic artery
9. 眶下动脉 infraorbital artery
10. 面横动脉 transverse facial artery
11. 上唇动脉 superior labial artery
12. 咬肌动脉 masseteric artery
13. 面动脉 facial artery
14. 下唇动脉 inferior labial artery
15. 颏动脉 mental artery

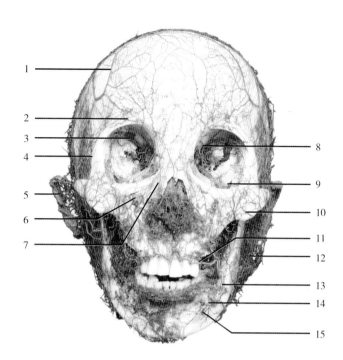

图1-3　头部血管（正面观）
the head vessels（frontal view）

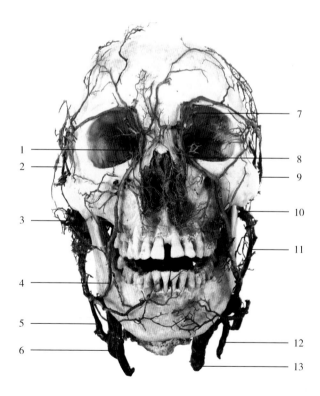

1. 眼下静脉 inferior ophthalmic vein
2. 颞浅静脉 superficial temporal vein
3. 翼静脉丛 pterygoid venous plexus
4. 面静脉 facial vein
5. 颈外静脉 external jugular vein
6. 颈内静脉 internal jugular vein
7. 眼上静脉 superior ophthalmic vein
8. 内眦静脉 angular vein
9. 颞浅静脉 superficial temporal vein
10. 上颌静脉 maxillary vein
11. 下颌后静脉 retromandibular vein
12. 颈外静脉 external jugular vein
13. 颈内静脉 internal jugular vein

图1-4　头面部静脉（正面观）
the veins of the head and face（frontal view）

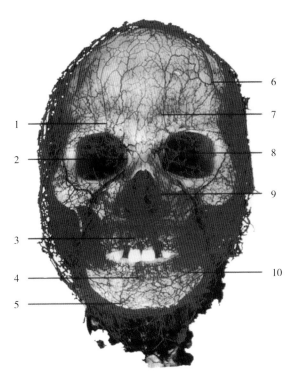

1. 眶上动脉 supraorbital artery
2. 内眦动脉 angular artery
3. 上唇动脉 superior labial artery
4. 下唇动脉 inferior labial artery
5. 颏下动脉 submental artery
6. 额支 frontal branch
7. 滑车上动脉 supratrochlear artery
8. 眼动脉 ophthalmic artery
9. 鼻外侧动脉 lateral nasal artery
10. 下唇动脉 inferior labial artery

图1-5 头颈部动脉铸型（前面观1）
the arterial cast of the head and neck（arterior view 1）

1. 颞动脉 temporal artery
2. 鼻背动脉 dorsal nasal artery
3. 鼻外侧动脉 lateral nasal artery
4. 面静脉 facial vein
5. 面动脉 facial artery
6. 额支 frontal branch
7. 眶上动脉 supraorbital artery
8. 内眦动脉 angular artery
9. 眶下动脉 infraorbital artery
10. 上唇动脉 superior labial artery
11. 下唇动脉 inferior labial artery

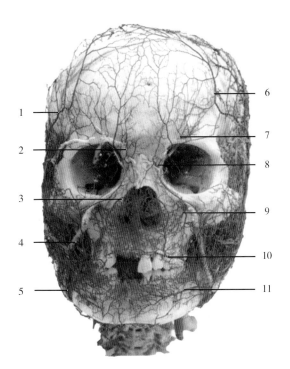

图1-6 头颈部动脉铸型（前面观2）
the arterial cast of the head and neck（arterior view 2）

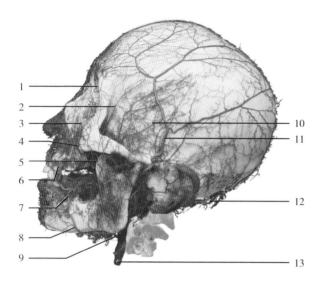

1. 眶上动脉 supraorbital artery
2. 颞深前动脉 anterior deep temporal artery
3. 内眦动脉 angular artery
4. 上牙槽前动脉 anterior superior alveolar artery
5. 冠突 coronoid process
6. 上唇动脉 superior labial artery
7. 下唇动脉 inferior labial artery
8. 面动脉 facial artery
9. 舌动脉 lingual artery
10. 颞深后动脉 posterior deep temporal artery
11. 颞浅动脉 superficial temporal artery
12. 枕动脉 occipital artery
13. 颈总动脉 common carotid artery

图1-7 头部血管（侧面观）
the head vessels（lateral view）

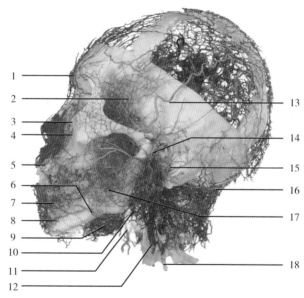

图1-8 头颈部动脉（侧面观）
the arteries of the head and neck（lateral view）

1. 眶上动脉 supraorbital artery
2. 颞深后动脉 posterior deep temporal artery
3. 内眦动脉 angular artery
4. 眶下动脉 infraorbital artery
5. 上唇动脉 superior labial artery
6. 面动脉 facial artery
7. 下唇动脉 inferior labial artery
8. 颏动脉 mental artery
9. 下颌下腺动脉网 submandibular gland artery network

10. 舌动脉 lingual artery
11. 咽升动脉 ascending pharyngeal artery
12. 颈外动脉 external carotid artery
13. 颞浅动脉 superficial temporal artery
14. 上颌动脉 maxillary artery
15. 耳后动脉 posterior auricular artery
16. 枕动脉 occipital artery
17. 咬肌动脉网 masseter artery network
18. 椎动脉 vertebral artery

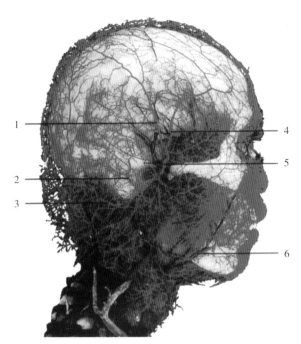

1. 顶支  parietal branch
2. 耳后动脉  posterior auricular artery
3. 枕动脉  occipital artery
4. 额支  frontal branch
5. 颞浅动脉  superficial temporal artery
6. 面动脉  facial artery

图1-9　头颈部动脉铸型（侧面观1）
the arterial cast of the head and neck（lateral view 1）

1. 顶支  parietal branch
2. 耳后动脉  posterior auricular artery
3. 枕动脉  occipital artery
4. 颞深前动脉  anterior deep temporal artery
5. 颞深后动脉  posterior deep temporal artery
6. 颞浅动脉  superficial temporal artery
7. 面横动脉  transverse facial artery
8. 面动脉  facial artery

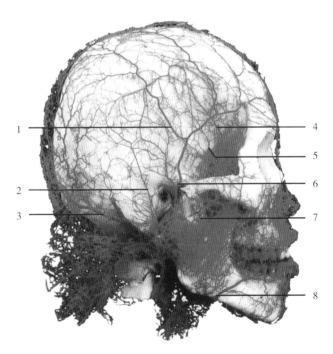

图1-10　头颈部动脉铸型（侧面观2）
the arterial cast of the head and neck（lateral view 2）

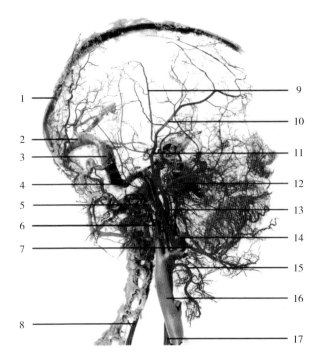

1. 上矢状窦 superior sagittal sinus
2. 横窦 transverse sinus
3. 乙状窦 sigmoid sinus
4. 耳后动脉 posterior auricular artery
5. 枕动脉 occipital artery
6. 胸锁乳突肌支 sternocleidomastoid branch
7. 舌动脉 lingual artery
8. 椎动脉 vertebral artery
9. 顶支 parietal branch
10. 额支 frontal branch
11. 颞浅动脉 superficial temporal artery
12. 上颌动脉 maxillary artery
13. 颈内动脉 internal carotid artery
14. 面动脉 facial artery
15. 甲状腺上动脉 superior thyroid artery
16. 颈内静脉 internal jugular vein
17. 颈总动脉 common carotid artery

图1-11　头颈部动脉铸型（侧面观3）
the arterial cast of the head and neck（lateral view 3）

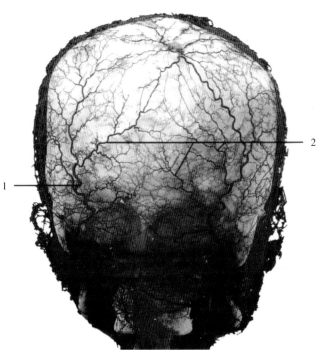

1. 枕动脉 occipital artery
2. 枕部动脉网 occipital artery network

图1-12　头面部动脉铸型（后面观）
the arterial cast of the head and face（posterior view）

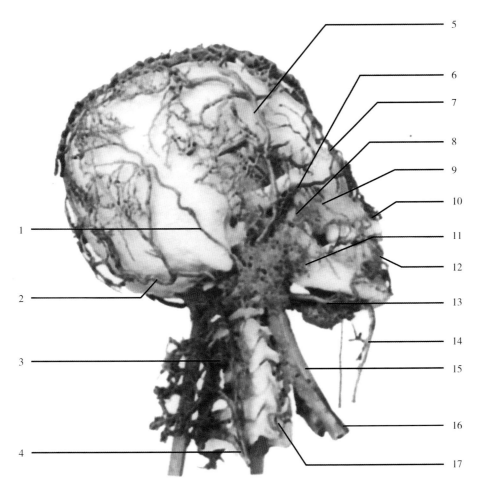

图1-13 头颈部静脉铸型（侧面观）
the renous cast of the head and neck （lateral view）

1. 耳后静脉 posterior auricular vein
2. 枕静脉 occipital vein
3. 椎外后静脉丛 posterior external vertebral venous plexus
4. 颈横静脉 transverse cervical vein
5. 颞浅静脉 superficial temporal vein
6. 面横静脉 transverse facial vein
7. 内眦静脉 angular vein
8. 翼静脉丛 pterygoid venous plexus

9. 上牙槽（后）静脉 posterior superior alveolar vein
10. 上唇静脉 superior labial vein
11. 面深静脉 deep facial vein
12. 下唇静脉 inferior labial vein
13. 面静脉 facial vein
14. 颈前静脉 anterior jugular vein
15. 颈外静脉 external jugular vein
16. 颈内静脉 internal jugular vein
17. 椎静脉 vertebral vein

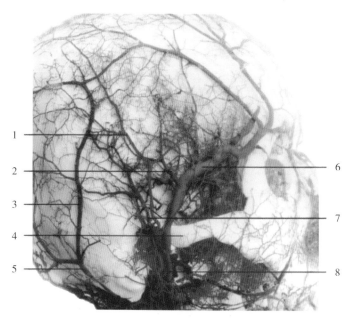

1. 顶支 parietal branch
2. 颞深静脉 deep temporal vein
3. 耳后静脉 posterior auricular vein
4. 颧弓 zygomatic arch
5. 枕静脉 occipital vein
6. 颞中静脉 middle temporal vein
7. 颞浅动、静脉 superficial temporal artery and superficial temporal vein
8. 下颌后静脉 retromandibular vein

图1-14 头面部动、静脉铸型（侧面观1）
the vessels cast of the head and face（lateral view 1）

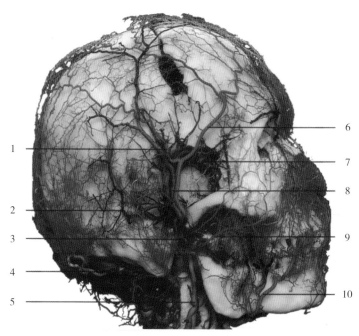

图1-15 头面部动、静脉铸型（侧面观2）
the vessels cast of the head and face（lateral view 2）

1. 顶支 parietal branch
2. 耳后静脉 posterior auricular vein
3. 下颌后静脉 retromandibular vein
4. 枕静脉 occipital vein
5. 颈外静脉 external jugular vein
6. 额支 frontal branch
7. 颞深动脉 deep temporal artery
8. 颞浅动、静脉 superficial temporal artery and superficial temporal vein
9. 面横动脉 transverse facial artery
10. 面动脉 facial artery

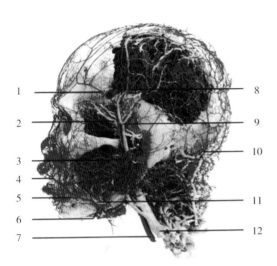

1. 额支 frontal branch
2. 颞中静脉 middle temporal vein
3. 腮腺动脉网 arterial network of parotid gland
4. 上唇动脉 superior labial artery
5. 下唇动脉 inferior labial artery
6. 面动脉 facial artery
7. 颈总动脉 common carotid artery
8. 顶支 parietal branch
9. 颞浅动、静脉 superficial temporal artery and superficial temporal vein
10. 枕动脉 occipital artery
11. 面静脉 facial vein
12. 颈内静脉 internal jugular vein

图1-16 头面部动、静脉铸型（侧面观3）
the vessels cast of the head and face
（lateral view 3）

1. 顶支 parietal branch
2. 颞中静脉 middle temporal vein
3. 颞浅静脉 superficial temporal vein
4. 枕动脉 occipital artery
5. 颈外静脉 external jugular vein
6. 额支 frontal branch
7. 颞浅动脉 superficial temporal artery
8. 翼静脉丛 pterygoid venous plexus
9. 下颌后静脉 retromandibular vein
10. 颈内静脉 internal jugular vein

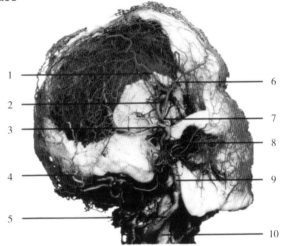

图1-17 头面部动、静脉铸型（侧面观4）
the vessels cast of the head and face（lateral view 4）

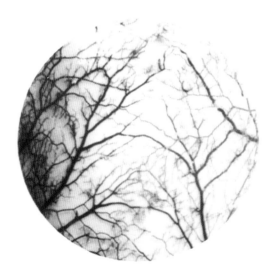

图1-18 头面部动、静脉铸型（顶面观）
the vessels cast of the head and face
（parietal view）

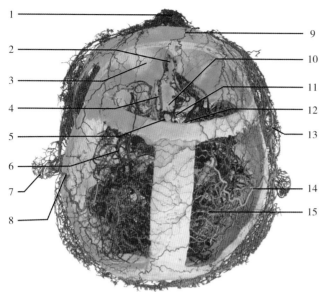

1. 鼻腭动脉 nasopalatine artery
2. 鸡冠 crista galli
3. 颅前窝 anterior cranial fossa
4. 大脑前动脉 anterior cerebral artery
5. 后交通动脉 posterior communicating artery
6. 颅中窝 middle cranial fossa
7. 耳动脉网 auricular artery rete
8. 颞浅动脉 superficial temporal artery
9. 眶上动脉 supraorbital artery
10. 大脑动脉环 cerebral arterial circle
11. 前交通动脉 anterior communicating artery
12. 大脑中动脉 middle cerebral artery
13. 颞浅动脉额支 frontal branch of superficial temporal artery
14. 颞浅动脉顶支 parietal branch of superficial temporal artery
15. 大脑后动脉 posterior cerebral artery

图1-19 头面部动脉（上面观）
the arteries of the head and face（superior view）

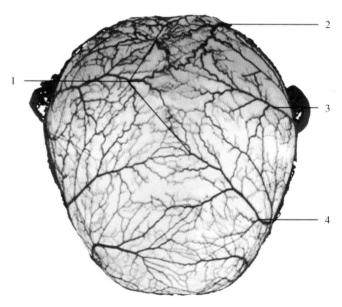

1. 顶部动脉网 parietal arterial rete
2. 左枕动脉 left occipital artery
3. 左顶支 left parietal branch
4. 左额支 left frontal branch

图1-20 头面部动脉铸型（顶面观）
the arterial cast of the head and face （parietal view）

1. 大脑上静脉 superior cerebral vein
2. 上矢状窦 superior sagittal sinus
3. 颈外静脉 external jugular vein
4. 耳后动、静脉 posterior auricular artery and posterior auricular vein
5. 枕动、静脉 occipital artery and occipital vein
6. 颈后静脉丛 retrojugular venous plexus

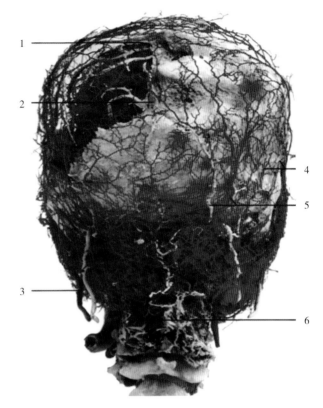

图1-21 头颈部动、静脉铸型（后面观）
the vessels cast of the head and neck （posterior view）

1. 板障 diploe
2. 板障管 diploic canals
3. 外板 outer plate

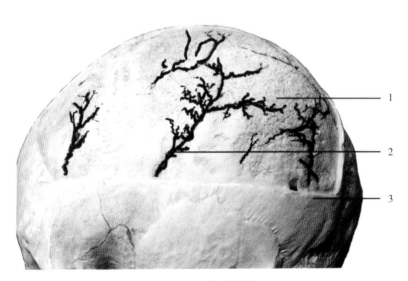

图1-22 板障静脉
the diploic veins

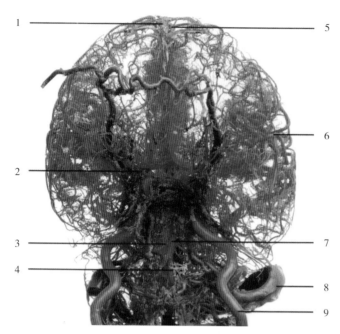

1. 上矢状窦 superior sagittal sinus
2. 眼动脉 ophthalmic artery
3. 小脑下前动脉 anterior inferior cerebellar artery
4. 椎动脉 vertebral artery
5. 大脑前动脉 anterior cerebral artery
6. 大脑中动脉 middle cerebral artery
7. 基底动脉 basilar artery
8. 乙状窦 sigmoid sinus
9. 颈内动脉 internal carotid artery

图1-23 大脑动脉铸型（前面观）
the cast of cerebral artery（arterior view）

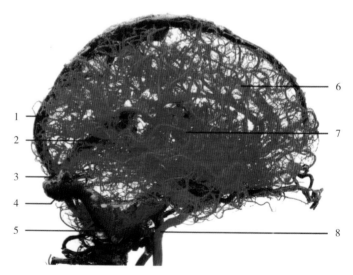

1. 上矢状窦 superior sagittal sinus
2. 下矢状窦 inferior sagittal sinus
3. 窦汇 confluence of sinuses
4. 横窦 transverse sinus
5. 乙状窦 sigmoid sinus
6. 大脑前动脉 anterior cerebral artery
7. 大脑中动脉 middle cerebral artery
8. 颈内动脉 internal carotid artery

图1-24 大脑动脉铸型（侧面观）
the cast of cerebral artery（lateral view）

1. 上矢状窦 superior sagittal sinus
2. 大脑上静脉 superior cerebral vein
3. 板障静脉 diploic vein
4. 大脑下静脉 inferior cerebral vein

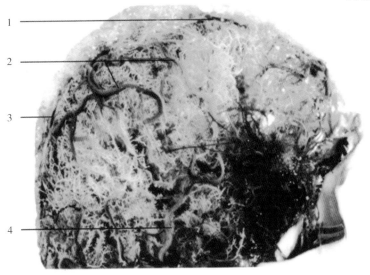

图1-25 大脑静脉铸型（侧面观）
the cast of cerebral vein（lateral view）

1. 大脑上静脉 superior cerebral vein
2. 大脑下静脉 inferior cerebral vein
3. 横窦 transverse sinus
4. 乙状窦 sigmoid sinus
5. 上矢状窦 superior sagittal sinus
6. 窦汇 confluence of sinuses

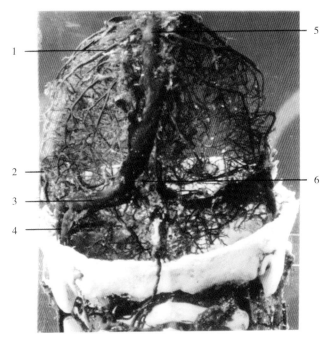

图1-26 大脑静脉铸型（后面观）
the cast of cerebral vein（posterior view）

1. 大脑上静脉 superior cerebral vein
2. 上吻合静脉 superior anastomotic vein
3. 横窦 transverse sinus
4. 大脑下静脉 inferior cerebral vein
5. 乙状窦 sigmoid sinus
6. 上矢状窦 superior sagittal sinus
7. 大脑中动脉 middle cerebral artery
8. 大脑中静脉 middle cerebral vein

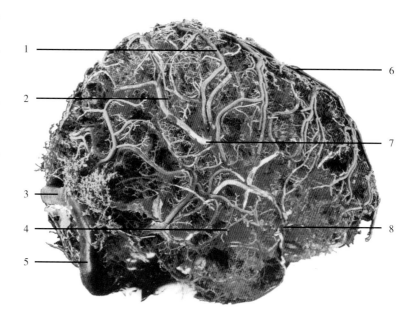

图1-27 大脑动、静脉铸型（侧面观）
the cast of cerebral artery and vein（lateral view）

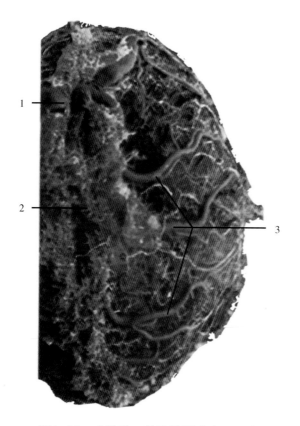

1. 上矢状窦 superior sagittal sinus
2. 蛛网膜颗粒 arachnoidal granulation
3. 大脑上静脉 superior cerebral vein

图1-28 大脑动、静脉铸型（上面观）
the cast of cerebral artery and vein（superior view）

1. 小脑上动脉 superior cerebellar artery
2. 小脑下动脉 anterior cerebellar artery
3. 椎动脉（寰椎部）vertebral artery（atlantic part）
4. 基底动脉 basilar artery
5. 椎动脉 vertebral artery

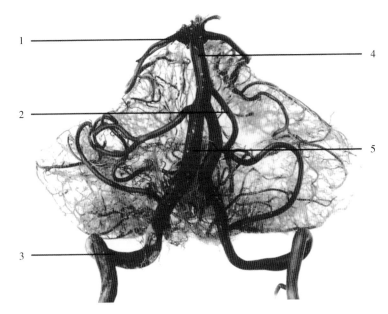

图1-29　小脑动脉铸型（前面观）
the cast of cerebellar arteries（anterior view）

1. 小脑上动脉 superior cerebellar artery
2. 基底动脉 basilar artery
3. 小脑下动脉 inferior cerebellar artery
4. 椎动脉（寰椎部）vertebral artery（atlantic part）

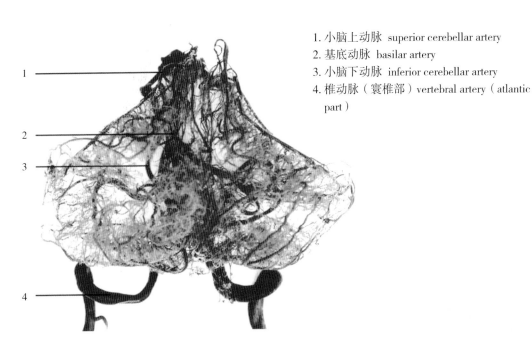

图1-30　小脑动脉铸型（后面观）
the cast of cerebellar arteries（posterior view）

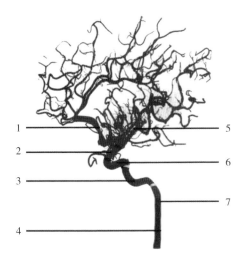

图1-31 颈内动脉铸型（内面观）
the cast of internal carotid artery
（internal view）

1. 大脑前动脉 anterior cerebral artery
2. 前床突上部 superior part of anterior clinoid process
3. 岩部 petrous part
4. 颈内动脉 internal carotid artery
5. 大脑中动脉 middle cerebral artery
6. 海绵窦部 cavernous part
7. 颈部 cervical part

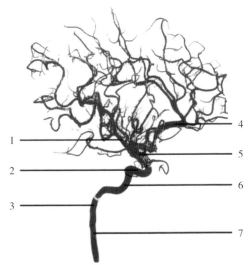

图1-32 颈内动脉铸型（外面观）
the cast of internal carotid artery
（external view）

1. 大脑中动脉 middle cerebral artery
2. 海绵窦部 cavernous part
3. 颈部 cervical part
4. 大脑前动脉 anterior cerebral artery
5. 前床突上部 superior part of anterior clinoid process
6. 岩部 petrous part
7. 颈内动脉 internal carotid artery

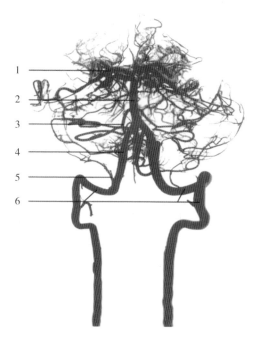

1. 小脑上动脉 superior cerebellar artery
2. 基底动脉 basilar artery
3. 小脑下前动脉 anterior inferior cerebellar artery
4. 椎动脉 vertebral artery
5. 小脑下后动脉 posterior inferior cerebellar artery
6. 椎动脉（寰椎部） vertebral artery（atlantic part）

图1-33 椎动脉铸型（前面观）
the cast of vertebral artery（anterior view）

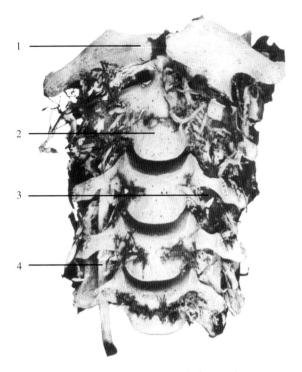

1. 寰椎 atlas
2. 枢椎 axis
3. 椎静脉 vertebral vein
4. 椎动脉 vertebral artery

图1-34 椎静脉铸型（前面观）
the cast of vertebral vein（anterior view）

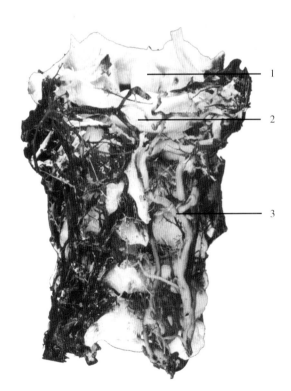

1. 齿突 dens
2. 寰椎 atlas
3. 颈后静脉丛 retrojugular venous plexus

图1-35 椎静脉铸型（后面观）
the cast of vertebral vein（posterior view）

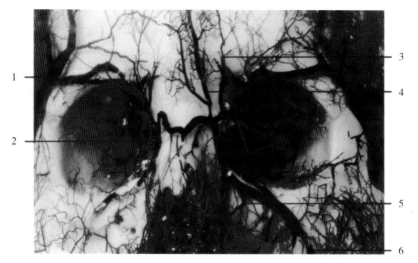

图1-36　眶部动、静脉铸型
the cast of orbital arteries and veins

1. 颞中静脉　middle temporal vein
2. 内眦静脉　venae angularis
3. 额动脉　frontal artery
4. 滑车上静脉　supratrochlear vein
5. 鼻外侧静脉　lateral nasal vein
6. 面静脉　facial vein

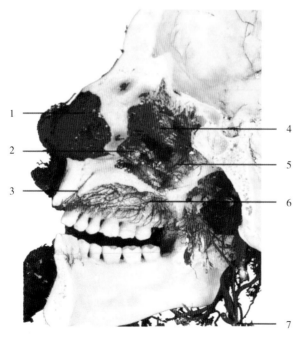

1. 鼻中隔动脉　nasalis septus artery
2. 下鼻甲动脉　inferior turbinate artery
3. 鼻腭动脉　nasopalatine artery
4. 中鼻甲动脉　middle turbinate artery
5. 鼻后外侧动脉　posterior lateral nasal artery
6. 腭大动脉　greater palatine artery
7. 颈外动脉　external carotid artery

图1-37　鼻腔内动脉铸型
the cast of internal nasal arteries

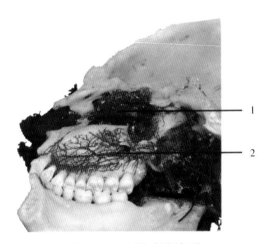

图1-38　上腭动脉铸型
the cast of palatal arteries

1. 鼻甲动脉 turbinate artery
2. 腭大动脉 greater palatine artery

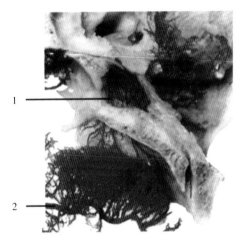

图1-39　舌动脉铸型（侧面观）
the cast of lingual artery（lateral view）

1. 腭降动脉 descending palatine artery
2. 舌动脉 lingual artery

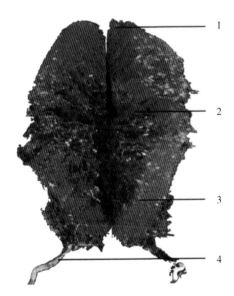

1. 舌尖动脉 apex lingual artery
2. 舌背动脉 dorsal lingual artery
3. 舌根动脉 radix lingual artery
4. 舌动脉 lingual artery

图1-40　舌动脉铸型（背面观）
the cast of lingual artery（dorsal view）

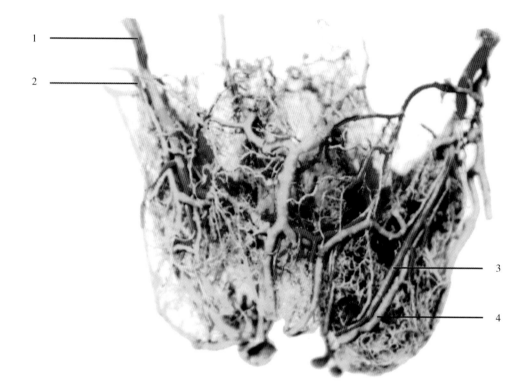

**图1-41　甲状腺血管铸型**
the cast of thyroid blood vessels

1. 甲状腺上动脉　superior thyroid artery
2. 甲状腺上静脉　superior thyroid vein
3. 甲状腺下动脉　inferior thyroid artery
4. 甲状腺下静脉　inferior thyroid vein

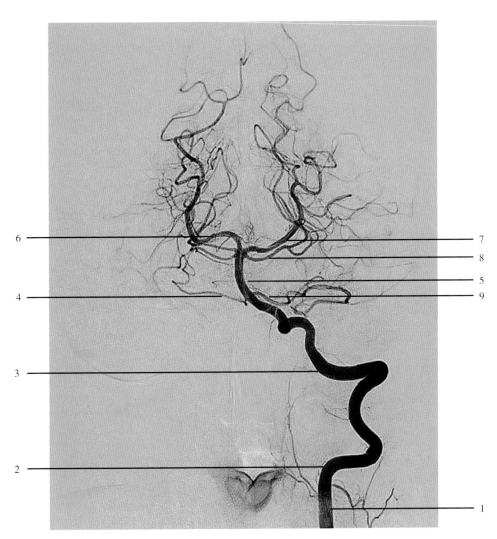

图1-42 椎基底动脉血管造影（正位）
the vertebral basilar artery angiography（pelvis）

1. 椎动脉 vertebral artery
2. 枢椎 axis
3. 寰椎 atlas
4. 右侧小脑下前动脉 right anterior inferior cerebellar artery（AICA）
5. 基底动脉 basilar artery
6. 右侧大脑后动脉 right posterior cerebral artery（PCA）
7. 左侧大脑后动脉 left posterior cerebral artery（PCA）
8. 左侧小脑上动脉 left superior cerebellar artery
9. 左侧小脑下前动脉 left anterior inferior cerebellar artery（AICA）

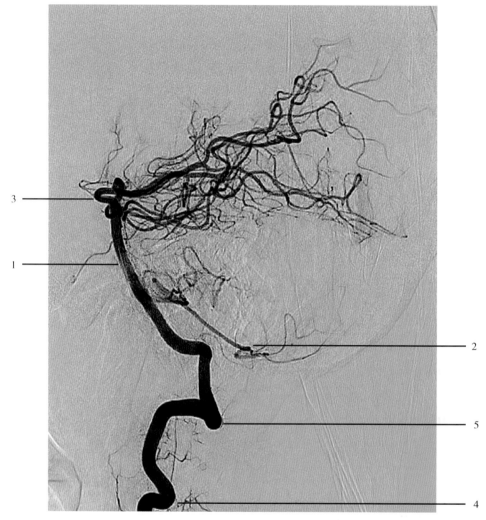

**图1-43 椎基底动脉血管造影（侧位）**
the vertebral basilar artery angiography（lateral position）

1. 基底动脉 basilar artery
2. 小脑下后动脉 posterior inferior cerebellar artery（PICA）
3. 大脑后动脉 posterior cerebral artery（PCA）
4. 寰椎 atlas
5. 枢椎 axis

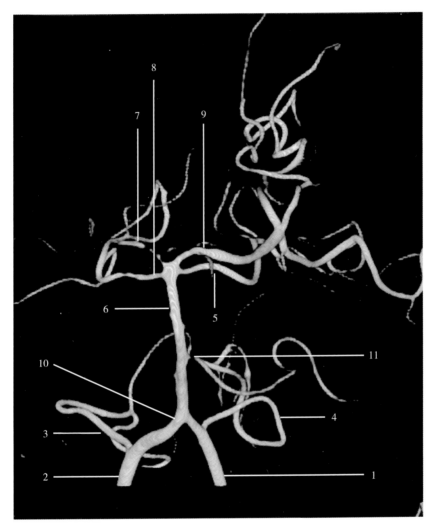

图1-44　椎基底动脉血管造影（3D）
the vertebral basilar artery angiography（3D）

1. 左侧椎动脉 left vertebral artery
2. 右侧椎动脉 right vertebral artery
3. 右侧小脑下后动脉 right posterior inferior cerebellar artery（PICA）
4. 左侧小脑下后动脉 left posterior inferior cerebellar artery（PICA）
5. 右侧小脑上动脉 right superior cerebellar artery
6. 基底动脉 basilar artery

7. 右侧大脑后动脉 right posterior cerebral artery（PCA）
8. 左侧小脑上动脉 left superior cerebellar artery
9. 左侧大脑后动脉 left posterior cerebral artery（PCA）
10. 椎基底动脉结合处 vertebral basilar junction
11. 小脑下前动脉 anterior inferior cerebellar artery（AICA）

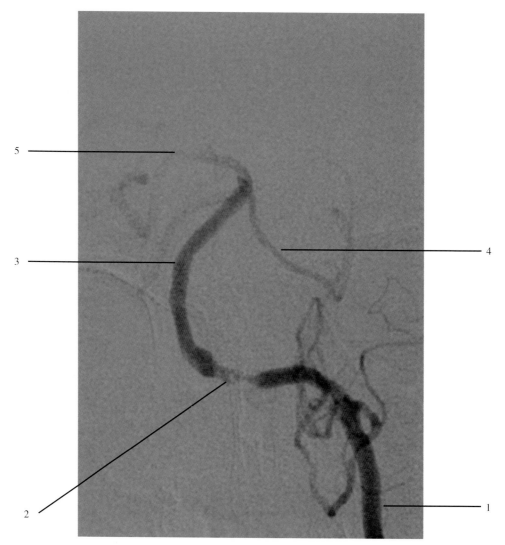

**图1-45　椎基底动脉狭窄**
vertebral basilar artery stenosis

1. 左侧椎动脉　left vertebral artery
2. 椎基底动脉狭窄　vertebral basilar artery stenosis
3. 基底动脉　basilar artery
4. 左侧小脑上动脉　left superior cerebellar artery
5. 右侧大脑后动脉　right posterior cerebral artery（PCA）

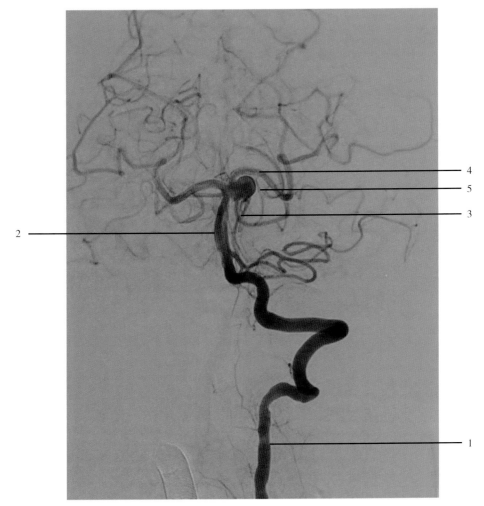

图1-46　左侧小脑上动脉动脉瘤
left superior cerebellar artery aneurysm

1. 左侧椎动脉　left vertebral artery
2. 基底动脉　basilar artery
3. 左侧小脑上动脉　left superior cerebellar artery
4. 左侧大脑后动脉　left posterior cerebral artery（PCA）
5. 左侧小脑上动脉动脉瘤　left superior cerebellar artery aneurysm（AN）

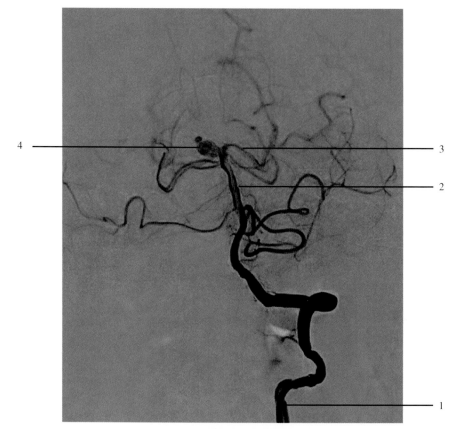

**图1-47 基底动脉尖动脉瘤**
basilar tip aneurysm

1. 左侧椎动脉 left vertebral artery
2. 基底动脉 basilar artery
3. 左侧大脑后动脉 left posterior cerebral artery（PCA）
4. 基底动脉尖动脉瘤 basilar tip aneurysm

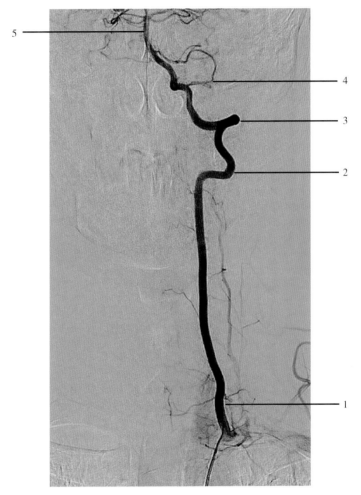

**图1-48　左侧椎动脉血管造影**
left vertebral artery angiography

1. 左侧椎动脉　left vertebral artery
2. 枢椎　axis
3. 寰椎　atlas
4. 小脑下后动脉 posterior inferior cerebellar artery（PICA）
5. 基底动脉　basilar artery

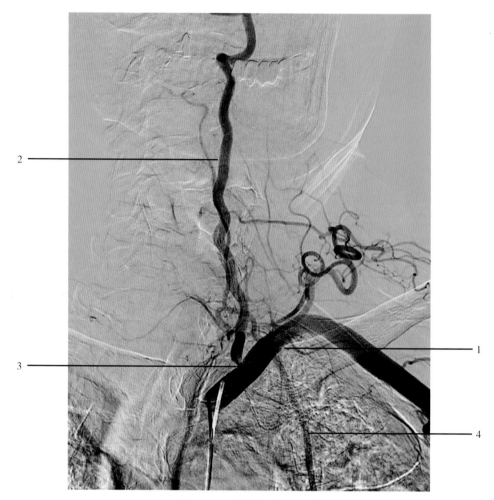

图1-49　左侧椎动脉狭窄
left vertebral artery stenosis

1. 左锁骨下动脉　left subclavian artery
2. 左侧椎动脉　left vertebral artery
3. 左侧椎动脉起始部重度狭窄　left vertebral artery severe stenosis
4. 左侧胸廓内动脉　left internal mammary artery

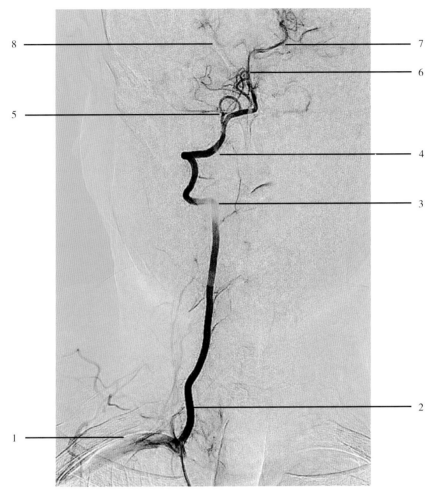

**图1-50　右侧椎动脉血管造影**
right vertebral artery angiography

1. 右锁骨下动脉　right subclavian artery
2. 右侧椎动脉　right vertebral artery
3. 枢椎　axis
4. 寰椎　atlas
5. 右侧小脑下后动脉　right posterior inferior cerebellar artery（PICA）
6. 基底动脉　basilar artery
7. 左侧大脑后动脉　left posterior cerebral artery（PCA）
8. 右侧大脑后动脉　right posterior cerebral artery（PCA）

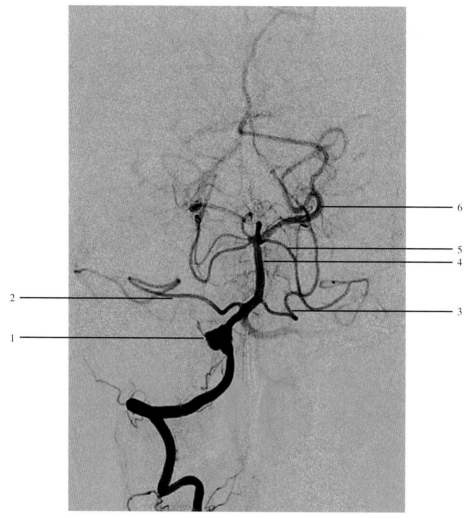

**图1-51 右侧椎动脉动脉瘤（正位）**
right vertebral artery aneurysm（pelvis）

1. 椎动脉解离性动脉瘤 vertebral artery dissociative aneurysm（AN）
2. 右侧小脑下前动脉 right anterior inferior cerebellar artery （AICA）
3. 左侧小脑下前动脉 left anterior inferior cerebellar artery （AICA）
4. 基底动脉 basilar artery
5. 左侧小脑上动脉 left superior cerebellar artery
6. 左侧大脑后动脉 left posterior cerebral artery（PCA）

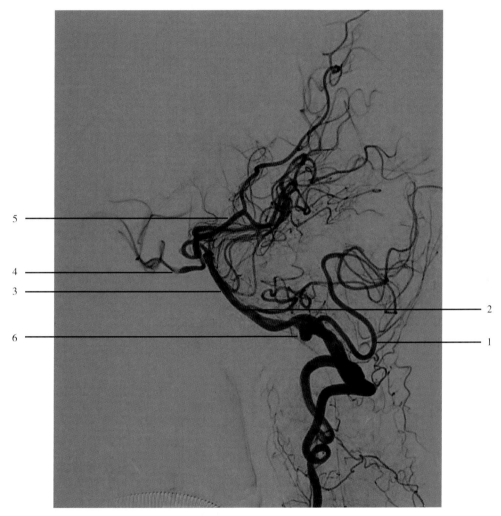

图1-52　右侧椎动脉动脉瘤（侧位）
right vertebral artery aneurysm（lateral position）

1. 小脑下后动脉 posterior inferior cerebellar artery（PICA）
2. 小脑下前动脉 anterior inferior cerebellar artery（AICA）
3. 基底动脉 basilar artery
4. 后交通动脉 posterior communicating artery
5. 大脑后动脉 posterior cerebral artery（PCA）
6. 椎动脉解离性动脉瘤 vertebral artery dissociative aneurysm（AN）

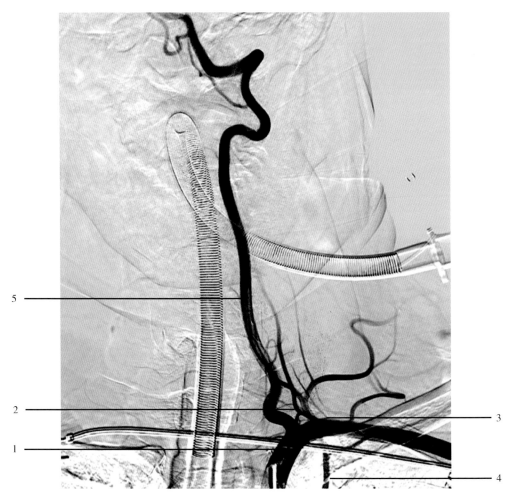

图1-53　左锁骨下动脉
left subclavian artery

1. 左锁骨下动脉　left subclavian artery
2. 左侧甲状颈干　left thyrocervical trunk
3. 左侧肋颈干　left costocervical trunk
4. 左侧胸廓内动脉　left internal mammary artery
5. 左侧椎动脉　left vertebral artery

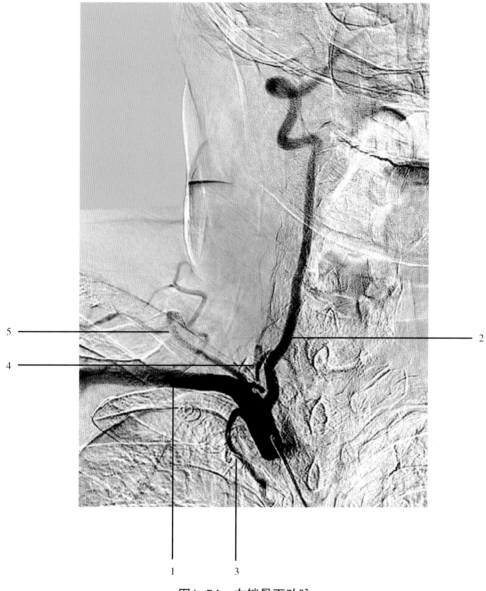

图1-54　右锁骨下动脉
right subclavian artery

1. 右锁骨下动脉　right subclavian artery
2. 右侧椎动脉　right vertebral artery
3. 右侧胸廓内动脉　right internal mammary artery
4. 右侧甲状颈干　right thyrocervical trunk
5. 右侧肋颈干　right costocervical trunk

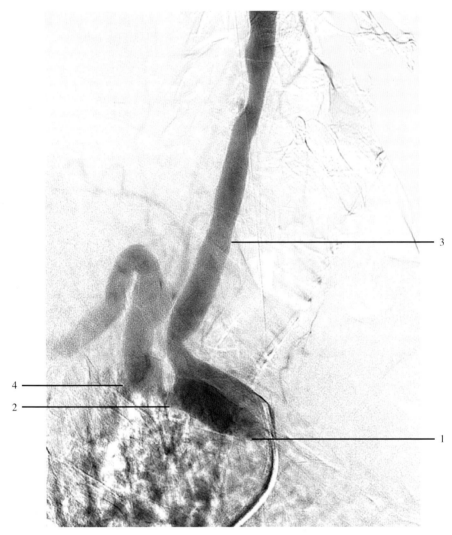

**图1-55　右锁骨下动脉重度狭窄**
right subclavian artery severe stenosis

1. 头臂干  innominate artery
2. 右锁骨下动脉  right subclavian artery
3. 右侧颈总动脉  right common carotid artery
4. 右侧锁骨下动脉重度狭窄  right subclavian artery severe stenosis

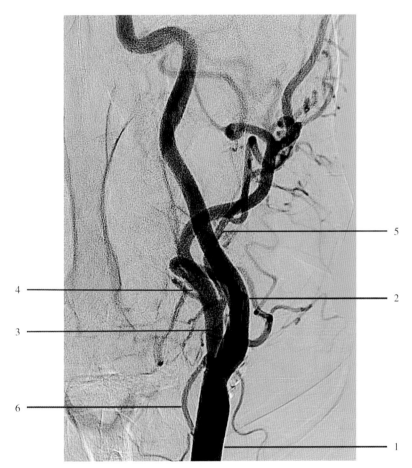

**图1-56 颈总动脉（正位）**
common carotid artery（pelvis）

1. 颈总动脉 common carotid artery
2. 颈内动脉 internal carotid artery
3. 颈外动脉 external carotid artery
4. 舌动脉 lingual artery
5. 枕动脉 occipital artery
6. 甲状腺上动脉 superior thyroid artery

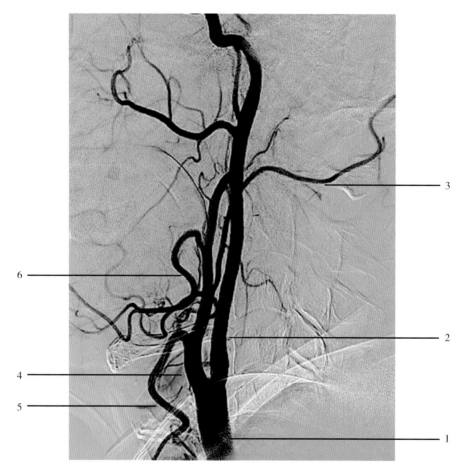

图1-57 颈总动脉（侧位）
common carotid artery（lateral position）

1. 颈总动脉 common carotid artery
2. 颈内动脉 internal carotid artery
3. 枕动脉 occipital artery
4. 颈外动脉 external carotid artery
5. 甲状腺上动脉 superior thyroid artery
6. 舌面动脉干 lingual-facial artery trunk

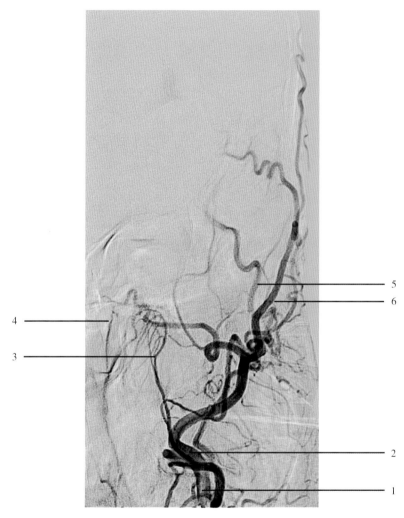

图1-58 颈外动脉（正位）
external carotid artery（pelvis）

1. 面动脉 facial artery
2. 枕动脉 occipital artery
3. 上颌动脉 maxillary artery
4. 蝶腭动脉 sphenopalatine artery
5. 脑膜中动脉 middle meningeal artery
6. 颞深动脉 deep temporal artery

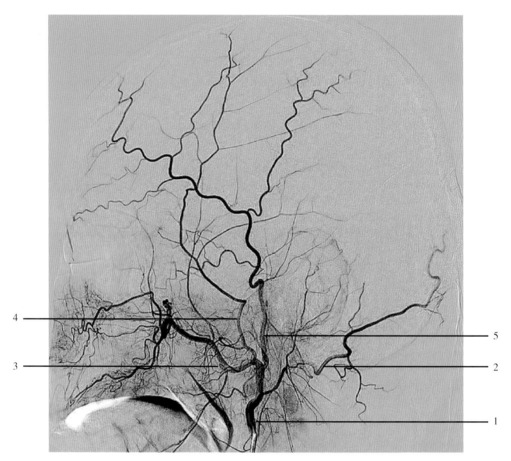

**图1-59　颈外动脉**
external carotid artery

1. 颈外动脉　external carotid artery
2. 枕动脉　occipital artery
3. 上颌动脉　maxillary artery
4. 脑膜中动脉　middle meningeal artery
5. 颞浅动脉　superficial temporal artery

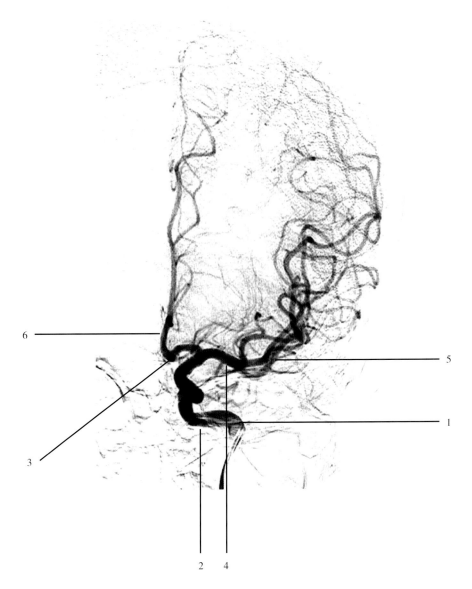

图1-60　左侧颈内动脉（正位）
left internal carotid artery（pelvis）

1. 颈内动脉-岩垂直段　internal carotid artery-vertical petrous segmen
2. 颈内动脉-岩水平段　internal carotid artery-horizontal petrous segment
3. 大脑前动脉A1段　A1 segment of anterior cerebral artery
4. 大脑中动脉M1段　M1 segment of middle cerebral artery
5. 大脑中动脉　middle cerebral artery
6. 大脑前动脉　anterior cerebral artery

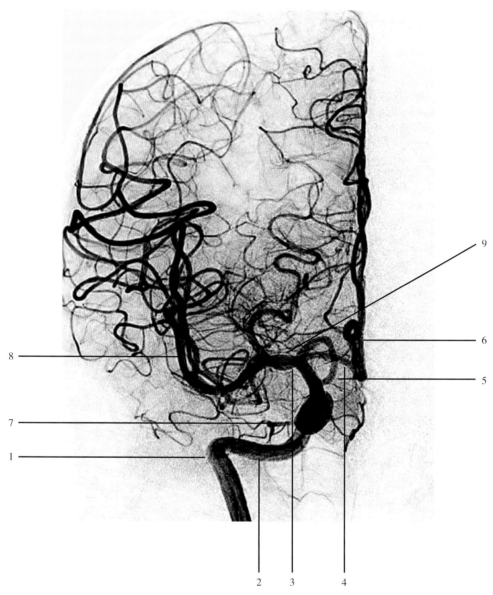

**图1-61　右侧颈内动脉（正位）**
right internal carotid artery（pelvis）

1. 颈内动脉-岩垂直段　internal carotid artery-vertical petrous segment
2. 颈内动脉-岩水平段　internal carotid artery-horizontal petrous segment
3. 颈内动脉分叉　internal carotid artery bifurcation
4. 大脑前动脉A1段　A1 segment of anterior cerebral artery
5. 后交通动脉　posterior communicating artery
6. 大脑前动脉　anterior cerebral artery
7. 眼动脉　ophthalmic artery
8. 大脑中动脉　middle cerebral artery
9. 大脑中动脉M1段　M1 segment of middle cerebral artery

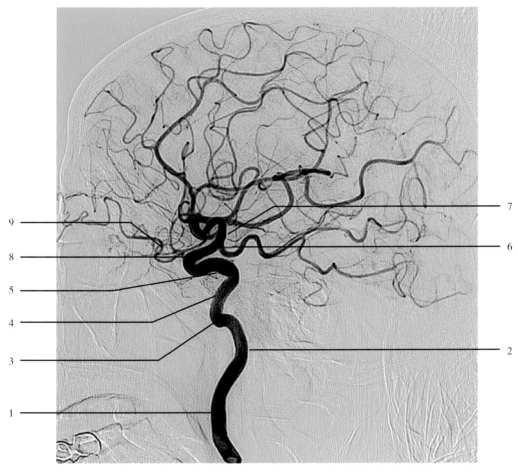

图1-62　颈内动脉（侧位）
internal carotid artery（lateral position）

1. 颈内动脉-颈段　internal carotid artery-cervical segment
2. 颈内动脉-岩垂直段　internal carotid artery-vertical petrous segment
3. 颈内动脉-岩水平段　internal carotid artery-horizontal petrous segment
4. 颈内动脉鞍前段　peresellar（Fisher C5）segment internal carotid artery
5. 颈内动脉海绵窦水平段　horizontal（Fisher C4）intracavernous segment internal carotid artery
6. 后交通动脉　posterior communicating artery
7. 颈内动脉床突上段　supraclinoid segment internal carotid artery
8. 颈内动脉海绵窦前膝段　anterior genu（Fisher C3）intracavernous segment internal carotid artery
9. 眼动脉　ophthalmic artery

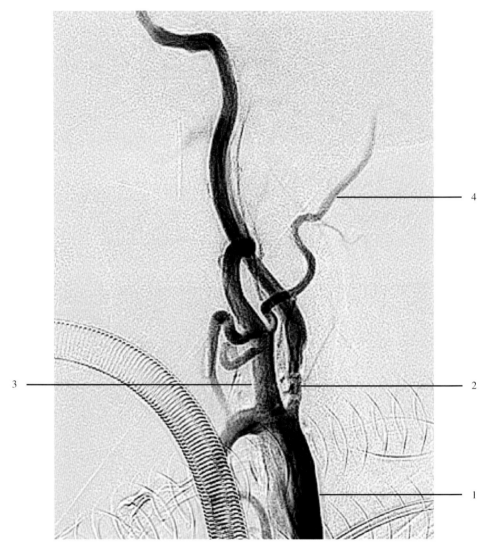

图1-63　颈内动脉狭窄
internal carotid artery stenosis

1. 颈总动脉　common carotid artery
2. 颈内动脉狭窄　internal carotid artery stenosis
3. 颈外动脉　external carotid artery
4. 枕动脉　occipital artery

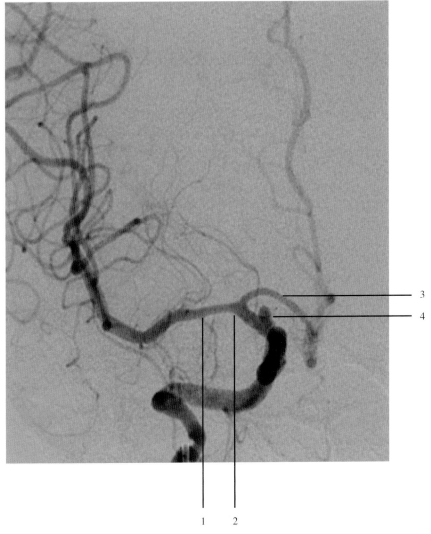

图1-64　血泡动脉瘤
blood blister-like aneurysm（BBA）

1. 大脑中动脉M1段　M1 segment of middle cerebral artery
2. 颈内动脉分叉　internal carotid artery bifurcation
3. 大脑前动脉A1段　A1 segment of anterior cerebral artery
4. 颈内动脉床突上段血泡样动脉瘤　Upper segment internal carotid artery blood blister-like aneurysm

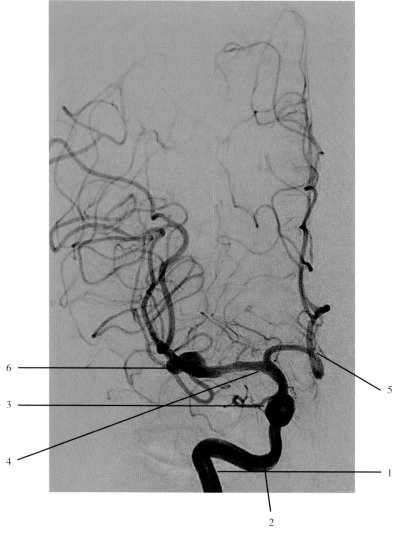

图1-65　大脑中动脉动脉瘤
middle cerebral artery aneurysm

1. 颈内动脉-岩垂直段　internal carotid artery-vertical petrous segment
2. 颈内动脉-岩水平段　internal carotid artery-horizontal petrous segment
3. 眼动脉　ophthalmic artery
4. 大脑中动脉M1段　M1 segment of middle cerebral artery
5. 大脑前动脉A1段　A1 segment of anterior cerebral artery
6. 右侧大脑中动脉分叉处动脉瘤　right middle cerebral artery bifurcation aneurysm

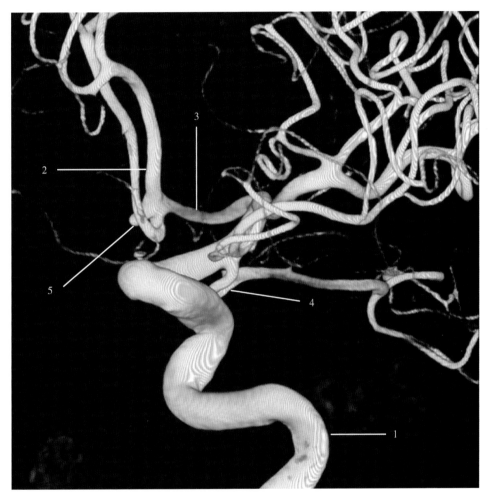

图1-66　前交通动脉动脉瘤
anterior commnicating artery aneurysm

1. 左侧颈内动脉　left internal carotid artery
2. 左侧大脑前动脉　left anterior cerebral artery
3. 左侧大脑前动脉A1段　left A1 segment of anterior cerebral artery
4. 后交通动脉　posterior communicating artery
5. 前交通动脉动脉瘤　anterior commnicating artery aneurysm

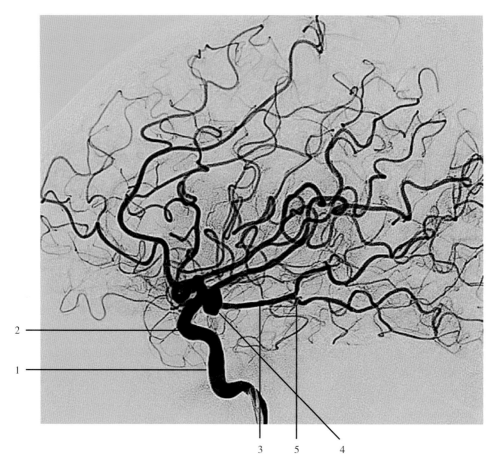

图1-67　后交通动脉动脉瘤
posterior communicating artery aneurysm

1. 颈内动脉鞍前段 peresellar（Fisher C5）segment internal carotid artery
2. 颈内动脉海绵窦前膝段 anterior genu（Fisher C3）intracavernous segment internal carotid artery
3. 后交通动脉 posterior communicating artery
4. 后交通动脉动脉瘤 posterior communicating artery aneurysm
5. 大脑后动脉 posterior cerebral artery（PCA）

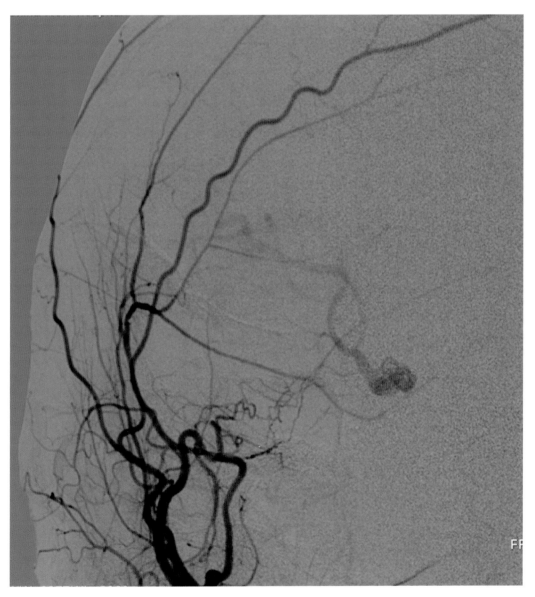

图1-68　海绵窦区硬脑膜动、静脉瘘（正位）
cavernous sinus dural arteriovenous fistula（pelvis）

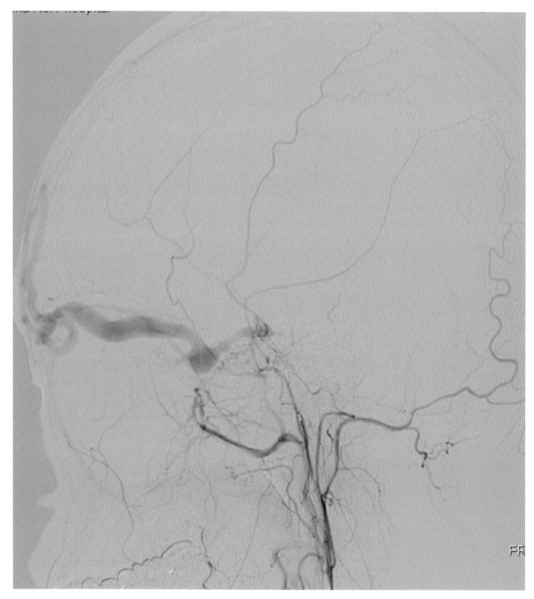

图1-69　海绵窦区硬脑膜动、静脉瘘（侧位）
cavernous sinus dural arteriovenous fistula（lateral position）

# 胸腹部血管

朱 巍 孙国生 王万粮

李 波 韩 建 东 洋

甄希成 李洪鹏

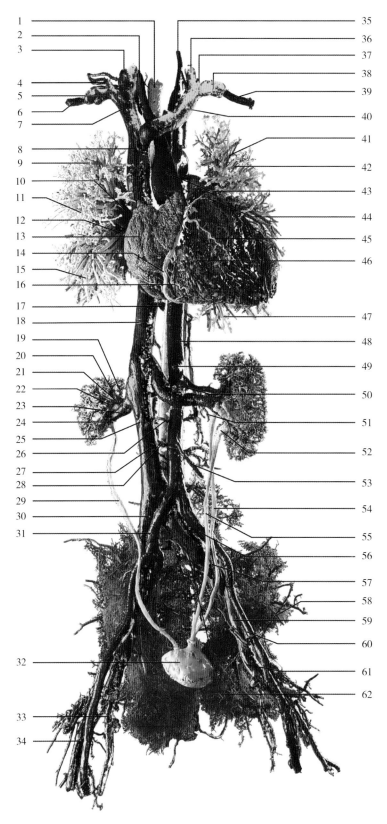

1
2
3
4
5
6
7
8
9
10
11
12
13
14
15
16
17
18
19
20
21
22
23
24
25
26
27
28
29
30
31
32
33
34

35
36
37
38
39
40
41
42
43
44
45
46
47
48
49
50
51
52
53
54
55
56
57
58
59
60
61
62

图2-1　胸腹器官联合铸型（后面观）
the cast of chest and abdomen（posterior view）

1. 气管 trachea
2. 头臂干 brachiocephalic trunk
3. 右颈内静脉 right internal jugular vein
4. 颈外静脉 external jugular vein
5. 右锁骨下静脉 right subclavian vein
6. 右锁骨下动脉 right subclavian artery
7. 右头臂静脉 right brachiocephalic vein
8. 上腔静脉 superior vena cava
9. 右肺上叶支气管 right superior lobar bronchus
10. 右肺上静脉 right superior pulmonary vein
11. 右肺中叶支气管 right middle lobar bronchus
12. 右肺下静脉 right inferior pulmonary vein
13. 右心房 right atrium
14. 右冠状动脉 right coronary artery
15. 右肺下叶支气管 right inferior lobar bronchus
16. 右冠状动脉心室支 right anterior ventricular branch
17. 肝静脉 hepatic vein
18. 下腔静脉 inferior vena cava
19. 上段动脉 superior segmental artery
20. 上前段动脉 superior anterior segmental artery
21. 肾动脉 renal artery
22. 下前段动脉 inferior anterior segmental artery
23. 肾动脉 renal artery
24. 下段动脉 inferior segmental artery
25. 右睾丸静脉 right testicular vein
26. 腰动脉 lumbar arteries
27. 下腔静脉 inferior vena cava
28. 腰静脉 lumbar vein
29. 输尿管 ureter
30. 髂总静脉 common iliac vein
31. 右髂总动脉 right common iliac artery
32. 膀胱 urinary bladder

33. 髂内静脉 internal iliac vein
34. 髂外静脉 external iliac vein
35. 左颈总动脉 left common carotid artery
36. 左颈内静脉 left internal jugular vein
37. 静脉角 venous angle
38. 左锁骨下静脉 left subclavian vein
39. 左锁骨下动脉 left subclavian artery
40. 左头臂静脉 left brachiocephalic vein
41. 左肺静脉 left pulmonary vein
42. 左肺上叶支气管 left superior lobar bronchus
43. 主动脉弓 aortic arch
44. 左室旋支 left anterior ventricular branch
45. 左冠状动脉前室间支 anterior interventricular branch of left coronary artery
46. 升主动脉 ascending aorta
47. 左肺下叶支气管 left inferior lobar bronchus
48. 腹主动脉 abdominal aorta
49. 腹腔干 celiac trunk
50. 肠系膜上动脉 superior mesenteric artery
51. 左睾丸静脉 left testicular vein
52. 肾盂 renal pelvis
53. 肠系膜下动脉 inferior mesenteric artery
54. 输尿管 ureter
55. 副输尿管 accessory ureter
56. 左髂总动脉 left common iliac artery
57. 髂内动脉 internal iliac artery
58. 旋髂动脉 iliac circumflex artery
59. 髂内静脉 internal iliac vein
60. 髂外动脉 external iliac artery
61. 腹壁下动脉 inferior epigastric artery
62. 髂总静脉 common iliac vein

1. 肺静脉 pulmonary vein
2. 肺动脉 pulmonary artery
3. 上腔静脉 superior vena cava
4. 右冠状动脉 right coronary artery
5. 主动脉弓 aortic arch
6. 肺动脉 pulmonary artery
7. 左冠状动脉 left coronary artery

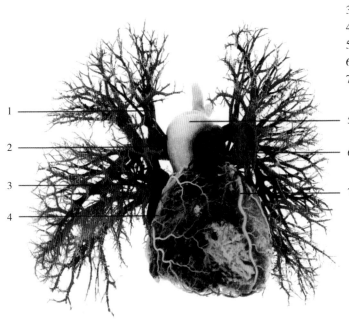

图2-2　心肺血管铸型（前面观1）
the cast of cardiopulmonary vessels （anterior view 1）

1. 肺静脉 pulmonary vein
2. 右心耳 right auricle
3. 右冠状动脉 right coronary artery
4. 主动脉弓 aortic arch
5. 肺动脉 pulmonary artery
6. 心大静脉 great cardiac vein
7. 左冠状动脉 left coronary artery

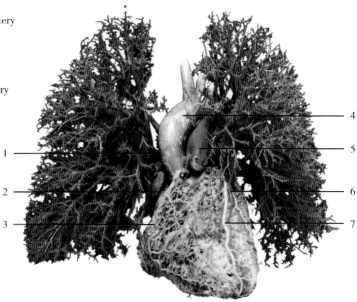

图2-3　心肺血管铸型（前面观2）
the cast of cardiopulmonary vessels （anterior view 2）

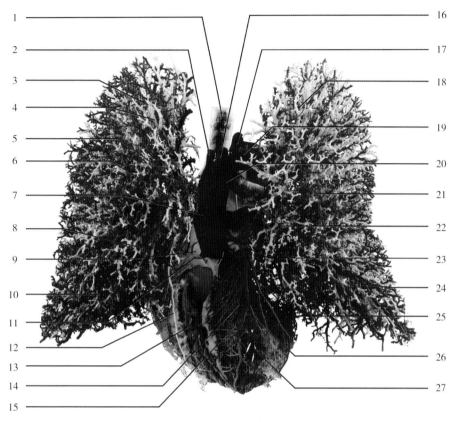

图2-4 心、肺（前面观）
heart and lung（anterior view）

1. 气管 trachea
2. 头臂干 brachiocephalic trunk
3. 上叶 superior lobe
4. 肺段支气管 segmental bronchi
5. 右肺上、下静脉 superior right pulmonary vein and inferior right pulmonary vein
6. 支气管 bronchi
7. 升主动脉 ascending aorta
8. 中叶 middle lobe
9. 窦房结支 branch of sinuatrial node
10. 右冠状动脉 right coronary artcry
11. 下叶 inferior lobe
12. 心大静脉 great cardiac vein
13. 右心室 right ventricle
14. 右室前支 anterior branch of right ventricle

15. 前室间支 anterior branch of interventricle
16. 左颈总动脉 left common carotid artery
17. 左锁骨下动脉 left subclavian artery
18. 上叶 superior lobe
19. 降主动脉 descending aorta
20. 主动脉弓 aortic arch
21. 肺段支气管 segmental bronchi
22. 左肺上、下静脉 superior left pulmonary vein and inferior left pulmonary vein
23. 左冠状动脉 left coronary artery
24. 对角支 diagonal branch
25. 下叶 inferior lobe
26. 左室前支 anterior branch of left ventricle
27. 左心室 left ventricle

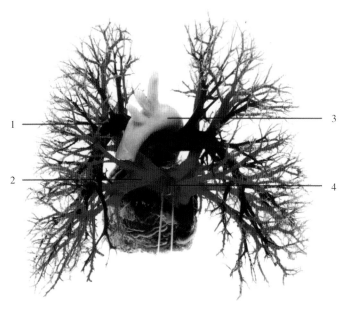

1. 肺动脉 pulmonary artery
2. 肺静脉 pulmonary vein
3. 主动脉弓 aortic arch
4. 左心房 left atrium

图2-5　心肺血管铸型（后面观）
the cast of cardiopulmonary vessels（posterior view）

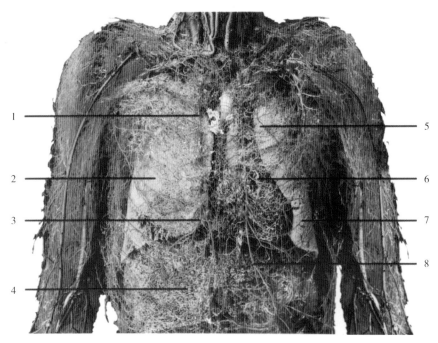

图2-6　心脏的位置（胸部铸型标本）
the position of heart（the cast of the thorax）

1. 胸廓内动脉 internal thoracic artery
2. 右肺 right lung
3. 肌膈动脉 musculophrenic artery
4. 肝 liver
5. 左肺 left lung
6. 心脏 heart
7. 肋间动脉 intercostal arteries
8. 腹壁上动脉 superior epigastric artery

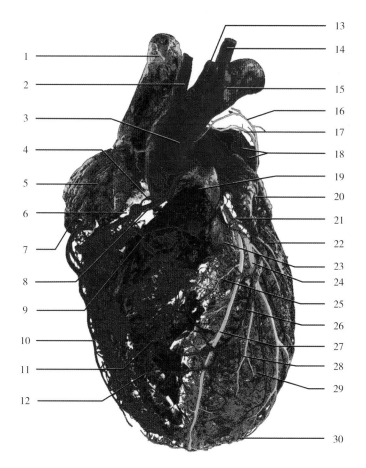

图2-7　心脏血管（右侧面观）
the cardial vessels（right lateral view）

1. 上腔静脉　superior vena cava
2. 头臂干　brachiocephalic trunk
3. 升主动脉　ascending aorta
4. 窦房结支　branch of sinuatrial node
5. 右心耳　right auricle
6. 右心房　right atrium
7. 右房支　right atrial branch
8. 右冠状动脉　right coronary artery
9. 右圆锥支　right conus branch
10. 右缘支　right marginal branch
11. 心前静脉　anterior cardiac vein
12. 右心室动脉　right ventricular artery
13. 左颈总动脉　left common carotid artery
14. 左锁骨下动脉　left subclavian artery
15. 主动脉弓　aortic arch

16. 左房旋支　left atrial circumflex branch
17. 窦房结支　branch of sinuatrial node
18. 肺静脉　pulmonary vein
19. 肺动脉干　pulmonary trunk
20. 左心耳　left auricle
21. 左冠状动脉　left coronary artery
22. 对角支　diagonal branch
23. 左圆锥支　left conus branch
24. 左室前支　anterior branch of left ventricle
25. 右室前支　anterior branch of right ventricle
26. 心大静脉　great cardiac vein
27. 前室间支　anterior branch of interventricle
28. 左室前支　anterior branch of left ventricle
29. 左心室　left ventricle
30. 心尖　cardiac apex

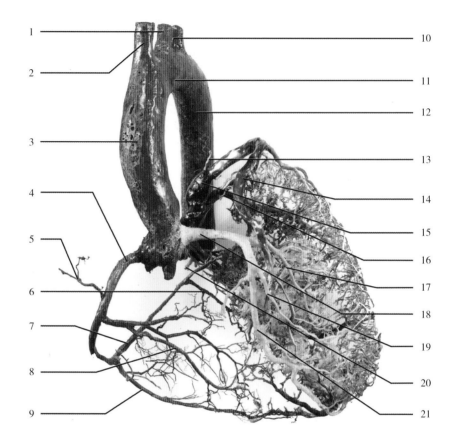

图2-8　心脏血管（主要显示室间隔供血）
the cardial vessels（showing the blood supply of interventricular septum）

1. 左颈总动脉　left common carotid artery
2. 头臂干　brachiocephalic trunk
3. 升主动脉　ascending aorta
4. 右冠状动脉　right coronary artery
5. 窦房结支　branch of sinuatrial node
6. 后室间支　posterior branch of interventricle
7. 右旋支　right circumflex branch
8. 右室前支　anterior branch of right ventricle
9. 右圆锥支　right conus branch
10. 右缘支　right marginal branch
11. 左锁骨下动脉　left subclavian artery

12. 降主动脉　descending aorta
13. 左心房斜静脉　oblique vein of left atrium
14. 心大静脉　great cardiac vein
15. 冠状窦　coronary sinus
16. 心中静脉　middle cardiac vein
17. 左室前支　anterior branch of left ventricle
18. 左冠状动脉　left coronary artery
19. 对角支　diagonal branch
20. 心小静脉　small cardiac vein
21. 前室间支　anterior branch of interventricle

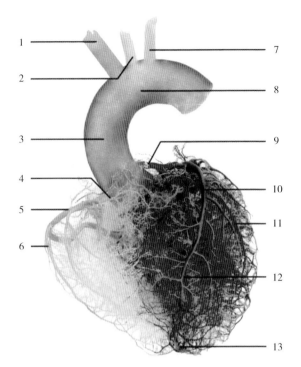

1. 头臂干　brachiocephalic trunk
2. 左颈总动脉　left common carotid artery
3. 升主动脉　ascending aorta
4. 动脉圆锥支　branch of arterial conus
5. 右冠状动脉　right coronary artery
6. 右缘支　right marginal branch
7. 左锁骨下动脉　left subclavian artery
8. 主动脉弓　aortic arch
9. 左冠状动脉　left coronary artery
10. 心大静脉　great cardiac vein
11. 左室前支　anterior branch of left ventricle
12. 前室间动脉　anterior interventricular artery
13. 心尖动脉　apical artery

图2-9　心脏血管铸型（前面观）
the cast of cardial vessels（anterior view）

1. 主动脉弓　aortic arch
2. 左冠状动脉　left coronary artery
3. 冠状窦　coronary sinus
4. 左室后静脉　posterior vein of left ventricle
5. 左缘支　left marginal branch
6. 升主动脉　ascending aorta
7. 右冠状动脉　right coronary artery
8. 右缘支　right marginal branch
9. 心中静脉　middle cardiac vein
10. 后室间支　posterior branch of interventricle

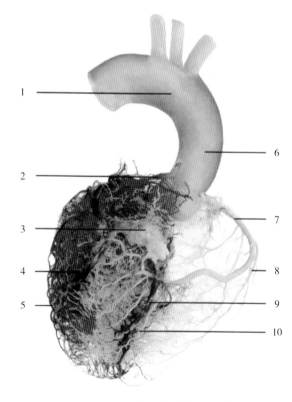

图2-10　心脏血管（底面观）
the cardial vessels（posterior view）

59

1. 左颈总动脉 left common carotid artery
2. 头臂干 brachiocephalic trunk
3. 升主动脉 ascending aorta
4. 右冠状动脉 right coronary artery
5. 右缘支 right marginal branch
6. 左锁骨下动脉 left subclavian artery
7. 主动脉弓 aortic arch
8. 左冠状动脉 left coronary artery
9. 旋支 circumflex branch
10. 左缘支 left marginal branch
11. 左室前支 anterior branch of left ventricle
12. 前室间支 anterior branch of interventricle

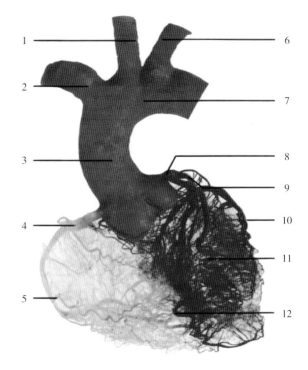

图2-11 心脏动脉分色铸型（前面观）
the dichroic cast of cardial artery（anterior view）

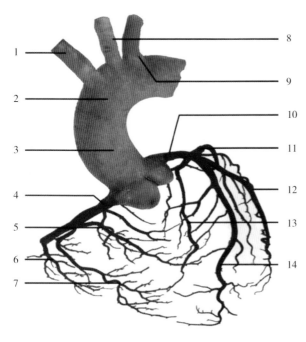

图2-12 心脏动脉铸型（前面观）
the cast of cardial artery（anterior view）

1. 头臂干 brachiocephalic trunk
2. 主动脉弓 aortic arch
3. 升主动脉 ascending aorta
4. 右冠状动脉 right coronary artery
5. 后室间支 posterior branch of interventricle
6. 右缘支 right marginal branch
7. 右室后支 posterior branch of right ventricle
8. 左颈总动脉 left common carotid artery
9. 左锁骨下动脉 left subclavian artery
10. 左冠状动脉 left coronary artery
11. 旋支 circumflex branch
12. 右室前支 anterior branch of right ventricle
13. 左室后支 posterior branch of left ventricle
14. 前室间支 anterior branch of interventricle

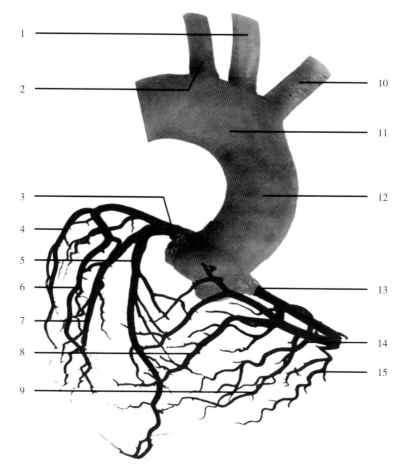

图2-13 心脏动脉铸型（后面观）
the cast of cardial artery（posterior view）

1. 左颈总动脉 left common carotid artery
2. 左锁骨下动脉 left subclavian artery
3. 左冠状动脉 left coronary artery
4. 左缘支 left marginal branch
5. 前室间支 anterior branch of interventricle
6. 左室后支 posterior branch of left ventricle
7. 左室前支 anterior branch of left ventricle
8. 后室间支 posterior branch of interventricle

9. 右室后支 posterior branch of right ventricle
10. 头臂干 brachiocephalic trunk
11. 主动脉弓 aortic arch
12. 升主动脉 ascending aorta
13. 右冠状动脉 right coronary artery
14. 右室前支 anterior branch of right ventricle
15. 右缘支 right marginal branch

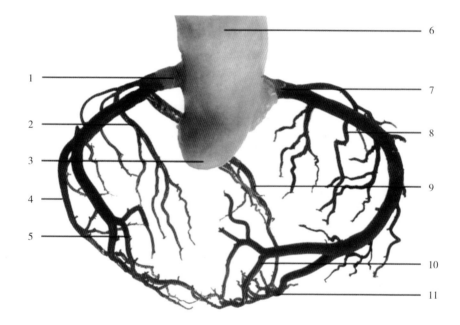

**图2-14　心脏动脉铸型（后上面观）**
the cast of cardial artery（supro-posterior view）

1. 左冠状动脉　left coronary artery
2. 左室前支　anterior branch of left ventricle
3. 后半月瓣　posterior semilunar valve
4. 左缘支　left marginal branch
5. 左室后支　posterior branch of left ventricle
6. 升主动脉　ascending aorta

7. 右冠状动脉　right coronary artery
8. 右室前支　anterior branch of right ventricle
9. 前室间支　anterior branch of interventricle
10. 后室间支　posterior branch of interventricle
11. 右室后支　posterior branch of right ventricle

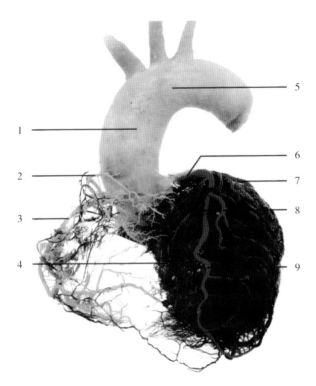

1. 升主动脉 ascending aorta
2. 动脉圆锥支 branch of arterial conus
3. 右冠状动脉 right coronary artery
4. 室间隔动脉 ventricular septal artery
5. 主动脉弓 aortic arch
6. 左冠状动脉 left coronary artery
7. 旋支 circumflex branch
8. 左室前支 anterior branch of left ventricle
9. 前室间支 anterior branch of interventricle

图2-15 心脏血管铸型（主要显示室间隔血供）
the cast of cardial vessels（showing the blood supply of interventricular septum）

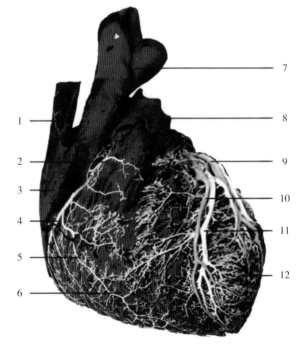

1. 上腔静脉 superior vena cava
2. 动脉圆锥支 branch of arterial conus
3. 右心房 right atrium
4. 右冠状动脉 right coronary artery
5. 右室前支 anterior branch of right ventricle
6. 右心室 right ventricle
7. 主动脉弓 aortic arch
8. 肺动脉 pulmonary artery
9. 左室前支 anterior branch of left ventricle
10. 前室间支 anterior branch of interventricle
11. 心大静脉 great cardiac vein
12. 左心室 left ventricle

图2-16 心脏血管、心腔铸型（前面观1）
the cast of cardial vessels and chambers（anterior view 1）

1. 动脉圆锥支 branch of arterial conus
2. 右室前支 anterior branch of right ventricle
3. 右冠状动脉 right coronary artery
4. 右缘支 right marginal branch
5. 右心室 right ventricle
6. 主动脉弓 aortic arch
7. 肺动脉 pulmonary artery
8. 左缘支 left marginal branch
9. 左室前支 anterior branch of left ventricle
10. 前室间支 anterior branch of interventricle
11. 左心室 left ventricle
12. 室间隔 interventricular septum

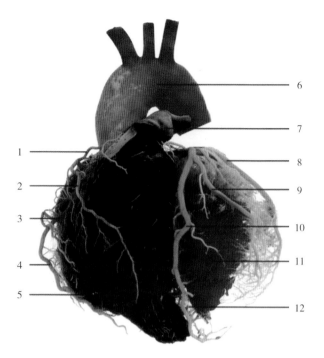

图2-17 心脏血管、心腔铸型（前面观2）
the cast of cardial vessels and cardial chambers
（anterior view 2）

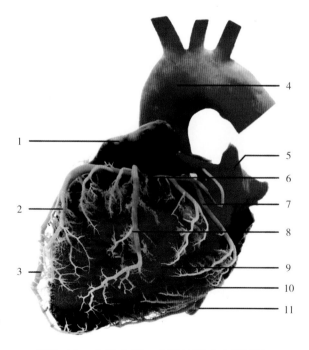

图2-18 心脏血管、心腔铸型（左面观）
the cast of cardial vessels and cardial chambers
（left view）

1. 肺动脉 pulmonary artery
2. 左室前支 anterior branch of left ventricle
3. 前室间支 anterior branch of interventricle
4. 主动脉弓 aortic arch
5. 左心房 left atrium
6. 左冠状动脉 left coronary artery
7. 旋支 circumflex branch
8. 左缘支 left marginal branch
9. 左心室 left ventricle
10. 左室后支 posterior branch of left ventricle
11. 后室间支 posterior branch of interventricle

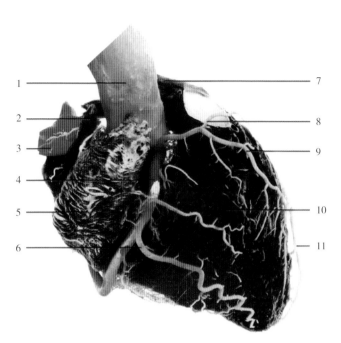

1. 升主动脉 ascending aorta
2. 上腔静脉 superior vena cava
3. 肺静脉 pulmonary vein
4. 右冠状动脉 right coronary artery
5. 右心房 right atrium
6. 右缘支 right marginal branch
7. 肺动脉 pulmonary artery
8. 动脉圆锥支 branch of arterial conus
9. 右室前支 anterior branch of right ventricle
10. 右心室 right ventricle
11. 前室间支 anterior branch of interventricle

图2-19 心脏血管、心腔铸型（右面观）
the cast of cardial vessels and cardial chambers
（right view）

1. 肺静脉 pulmonary vein
2. 左心房 left atrium
3. 旋支 circumflex branch
4. 左缘支 left marginal branch
5. 左心室 left ventricle
6. 室间隔 interventricular septum
7. 主动脉弓 aortic arch
8. 升主动脉 ascending aorta
9. 右心房 right atrium
10. 右冠状动脉 right coronary artery
11. 后室间支 posterior branch of interventricle
12. 右心室 right ventricle

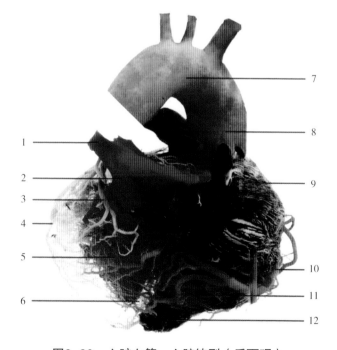

图2-20 心脏血管、心腔铸型（后面观）
the cast of cardial vessels and cardial chambers
（posterior view）

1. 升主动脉 ascending aorta
2. 动脉圆锥支 branch of arterial conus
3. 右冠状动脉 right coronary artery
4. 心前静脉 anterior cardial vein
5. 心小静脉 small cardiac vein
6. 心大静脉 great cardiac vein
7. 左室前支 anterior branch of left ventricle
8. 前室间支 anterior branch of interventricle

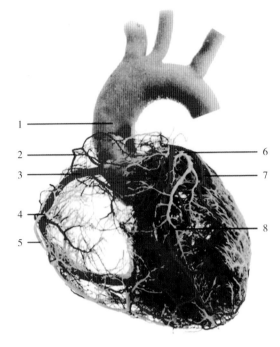

图2-21　心脏血管铸型（前面观）
the cast of cardial vessels（anterior view）

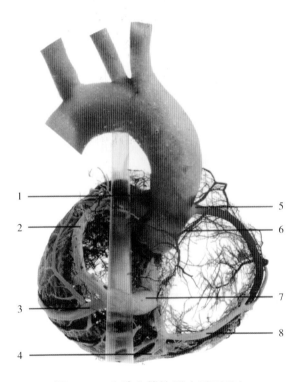

图2-22　心脏血管铸型（后面观）
the cast of cardial vessels（posterior view）

1. 左冠状动脉 left coronary artery
2. 心大静脉 great cardiac vein
3. 左室后静脉 posterior vein of left ventricle
4. 心中静脉 middle cardiac vein
5. 右冠状动脉 right coronary artery
6. 室间隔支 interventricular septum branch
7. 冠状窦 coronary sinus
8. 心小静脉 small cardiac vein

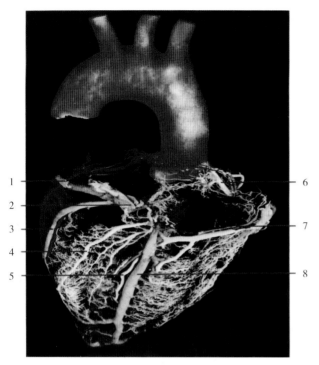

1. 心大静脉 great cardiac vein
2. 冠状窦 coronary sinus
3. 左室后静脉 posterior vein of left ventricle
4. 左室后支 posterior branch of left ventricle
5. 后室间支 posterior branch of interventricle
6. 右冠状动脉 right coronary artery
7. 心小静脉 small cardiac vein
8. 心中静脉 middle cardiac vein

图2-23　心脏血管铸型（膈面观）
the cast of cardial vessels（diaphragmatical view）

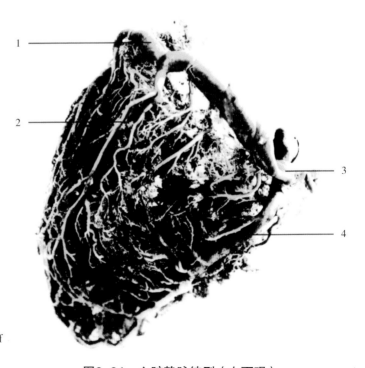

1. 心大静脉 great cardiac vein
2. 左室后静脉 posterior vein of left ventricle
3. 冠状窦 coronary sinus
4. 心中静脉 middle cardiac vein

图2-24　心脏静脉铸型（左面观）
the cast of cardial veins（left view）

1. 心大静脉 great cardiac vein
2. 冠状窦 coronary sinus
3. 心小静脉 small cardiac vein
4. 心大静脉 great cardiac vein
5. 右冠状动脉 right coronary artery
6. 心前静脉 anterior cardiac vein

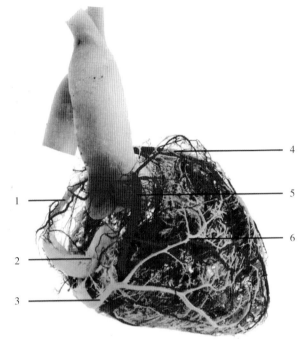

图2-25 心脏静脉铸型（右面观）
the cast of cardial veins（right view）

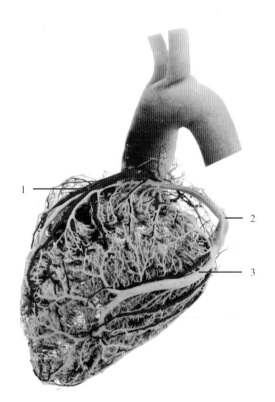

1. 前室间支 anterior branch of interventricle
2. 心大静脉 great cardiac vein
3. 心中静脉 middle cardiac vein

图2-26 心脏动、静脉铸型（左面观）
the cast of cardial arteries and veins（left view）

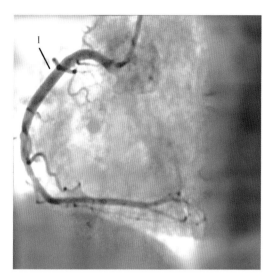

右冠状动脉造影（左前斜位41°）

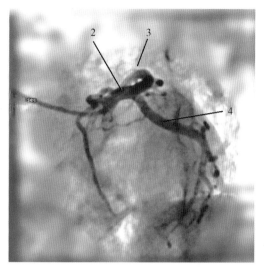

左冠状动脉造影（左前斜位48°+足位30°）

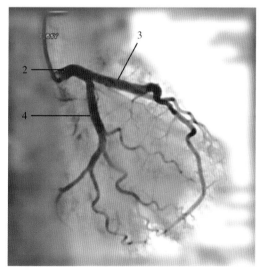

左冠状动脉造影（右前斜位27°+足位25°）

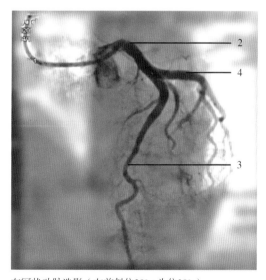

左冠状动脉造影（左前斜位28°+头位28°）

图2-27　正常冠状动脉造影像
normal coronary artery angiography

1. RCA　　2. LM　　3. LAD　　4. LCX

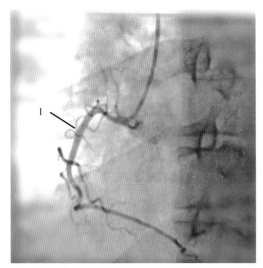

右冠状动脉造影（左前斜位38°）

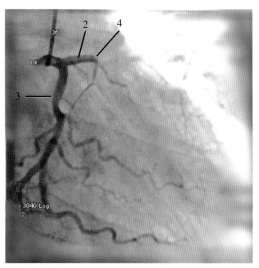

左冠状动脉造影（右前斜位26°＋足位25°）

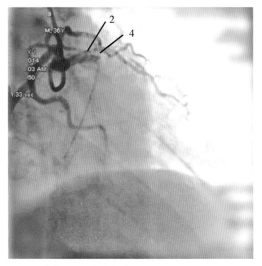

左冠状动脉造影（右前斜位34°）

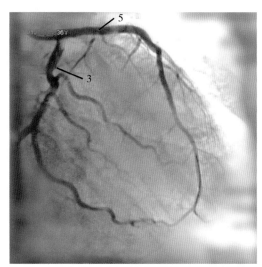

左冠状动脉造影（右前斜位41°＋足位28°）

图2-28　急性前壁心肌梗死+LAD PCI术
acute anterior myocardial infarction+LCX PCI

1. RCA
2. LAD
3. LCX
4. LAD中段100%闭塞
5. LAD中段闭塞支架术后远端血管显影

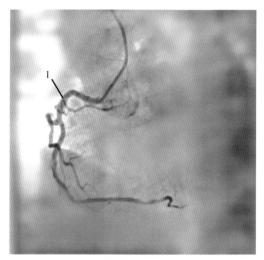

右冠状动脉造影（左前斜位42°）

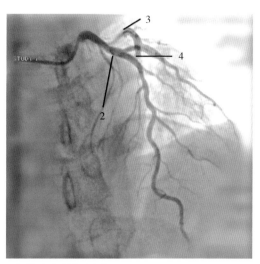

左冠状动脉造影（头位25°）

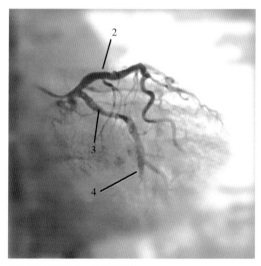

左冠状动脉造影（右前斜位30°）

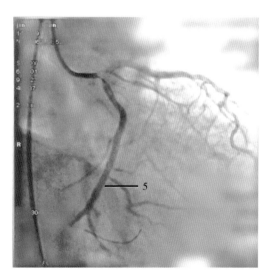

左冠状动脉造影（右前斜位31°＋足位29°）

图2-29 急性下壁心肌梗死+LCX PCI术
acute inferior myocardial infarction+LCX PCI

1. RCA
2. LAD
3. LCX
4. LCX中段以远完全闭塞
5. LCX闭塞处行支架，术后远端血管显影

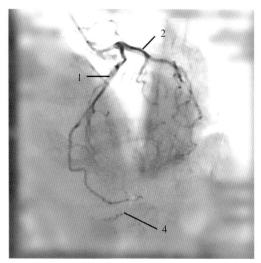

左冠状动脉造影（头位25°）

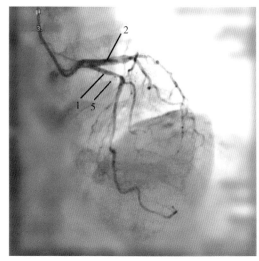

左冠状动脉造影（头位25°）

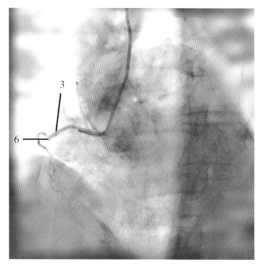

左冠状动脉造影（头位25°）

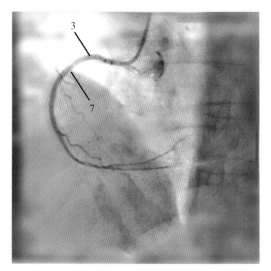

左冠状动脉造影（头位25°）

图2-30　急性下壁心肌梗死+RCA PCI术
acute inferior myocardial infarction+RCA PCI

1. LAD
2. LCX
3. RCA
4. 左冠脉给右冠脉远端提供侧支循环
5. LAD近段50%狭窄
6. RCA中段100%闭塞
7. RCA闭塞处支架术后，远端血管显影

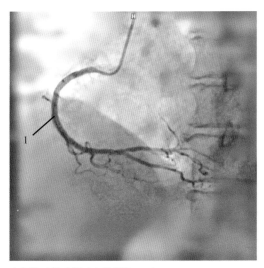

右冠状动脉造影（左前斜位37°）

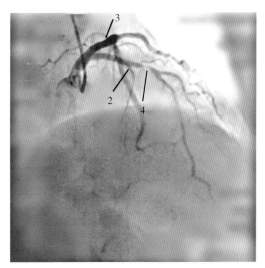

左冠状动脉造影（右前斜位30°+头位27°）

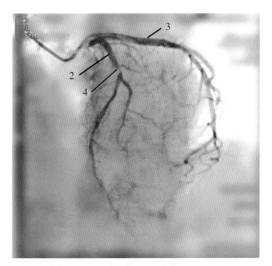

左冠状动脉造影（左前斜位28°+头位27°）

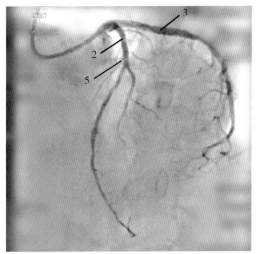

左冠状动脉造影（左前斜位35°+头位30°）

**图2-31　急性非ST段抬高型心肌梗死+LAD PCI术**
acute non ST segment elevation myocardial infarction+LAD PCI

1. RCA
2. LAD
3. LCX
4. LAD中段90%狭窄
5. LAD中段行支架术后，无残余狭窄

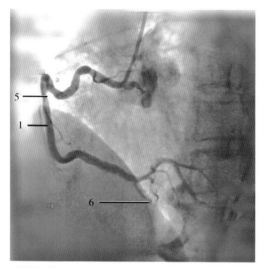

右冠状动脉造影（左前斜位38°）

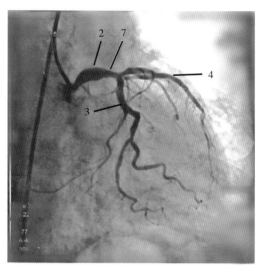

左冠状动脉造影（右前斜位30°+足位20°）

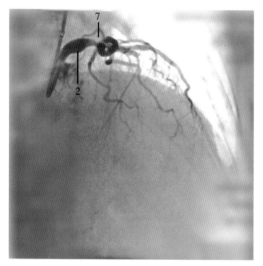

左冠状动脉造影（右前斜位27°+头位25°）

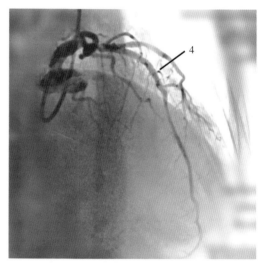

左冠状动脉造影（右前斜位37°+头位28°）

图2-32　不稳定型心绞痛（1）
unstable angina（1）

1. RCA
2. LM
3. LCX
4. LAD
5. RCA中段80%狭窄
6. RCA远端闭塞
7. LM远段60%狭窄

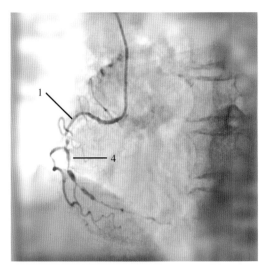

右冠状动脉造影（左前斜位39°）

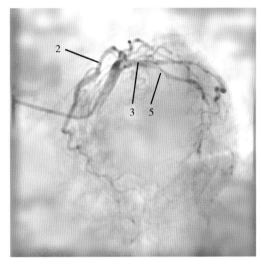

左冠状动脉造影（右前斜位40°+头位29°）

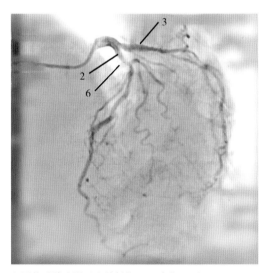

左冠状动脉造影（左前斜位30°+头位28°）

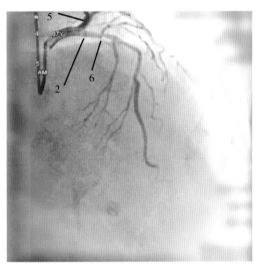

左冠状动脉造影（右前斜位31°+头位28°）

**图2-33　不稳定型心绞痛（2）**
unstable angina（2）

1. RCA
2. LAD
3. LCX
4. RCA近中段弥漫性病变狭窄伴远端完全闭塞
5. LCX中段50%狭窄
6. LAD近段70%狭窄

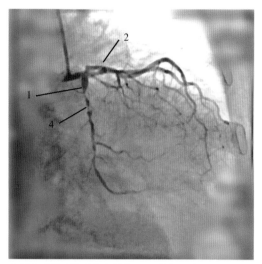

左冠状动脉造影（右前斜位29°＋足位23°）

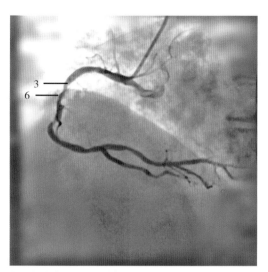

右冠状动脉造影（左前斜位43°）

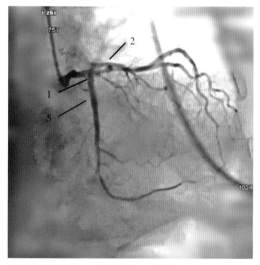

左冠状动脉造影（右前斜位30°＋足位27°）

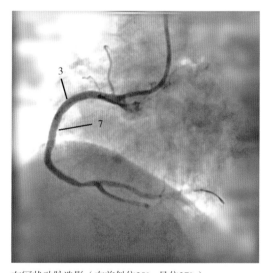

左冠状动脉造影（右前斜位30°＋足位27°）

**图2-34 不稳定型心绞痛+RCA PCI术（1）**
unstable angina+RCA PCI（1）

1. LCX
2. LAD
3. RCA
4. LCX近中段70%狭窄
5. LCX病变支架术后
6. RCA中段60%～75%狭窄
7. RCA中段病变支架术后

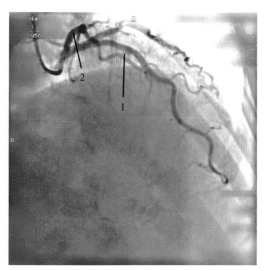

左冠状动脉造影（右前斜位39°＋头位30°）

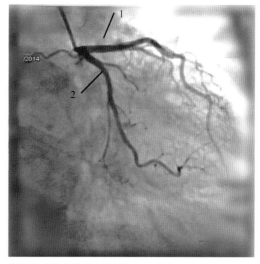

左冠状动脉造影（右前斜位29°＋足位24°）

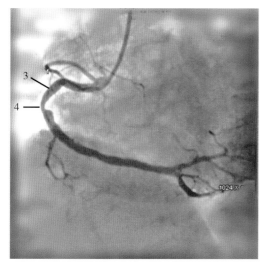

右冠状动脉造影（左前斜位43°）

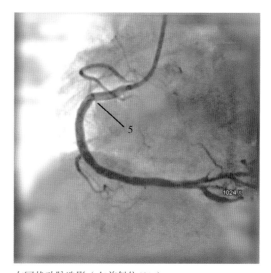

右冠状动脉造影（左前斜位42°）

图2-35　不稳定型心绞痛+RCA PCI术（2）
unstable angina+RCA PCI（2）

1. LAD
2. LCX
3. RCA
4. RCA中段75%狭窄
5. RCA病变支架术后

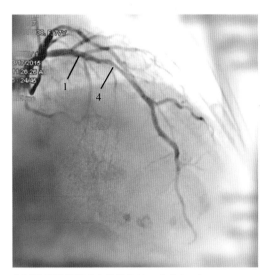
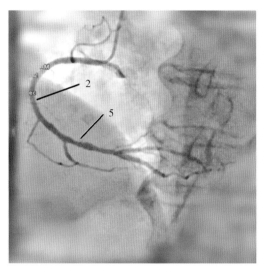

左冠状动脉造影（右前斜位29°+头位29°）　　　右冠状动脉造影（左前斜位39°）

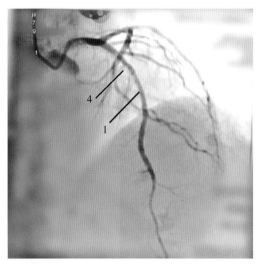
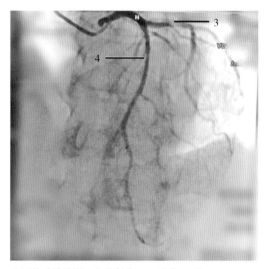

左冠状动脉造影（左前斜位3°+头位32°）　　　左冠状动脉造影（左前斜位29°+头位31°）

**图2-36　冠状动脉粥样硬化**
atherosclerosis

1. LAD
2. RCA
3. LCX
4. LAD中段40%狭窄
5. RCA远段30%狭窄，药物保守治疗，未行支架术

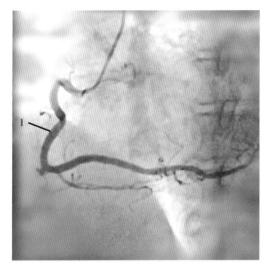
右冠状动脉造影（左前斜位39°）

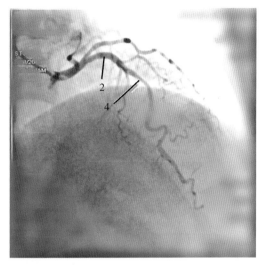
左冠状动脉造影（右前斜位39°+头位31°）

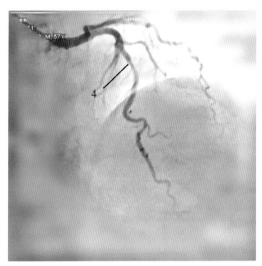
左冠状动脉造影（头位31°）

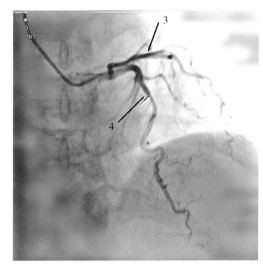
左冠状动脉造影（头位28°）

**图2-37　冠心病稳定型心绞痛**
coronary heart disease stable angina

1. RCA
2. LAD
3. LCX
4. LAD中段50%狭窄。轻度病变药物保守治疗，未行支架术

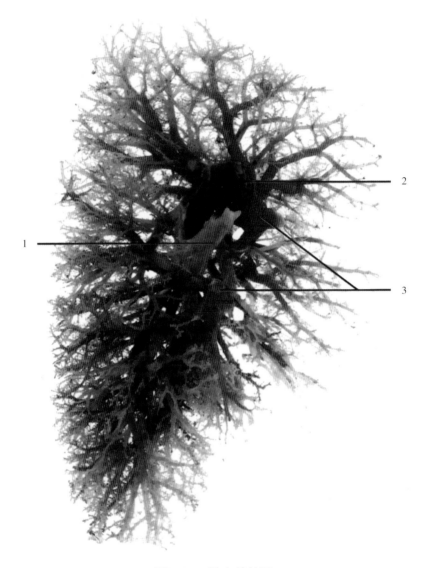

图2-38　肺血管铸型
the cast of pulmonary vessels

1. 支气管　bronchi
2. 肺动脉　pulmonary artery
3. 肺静脉　pulmonary vein

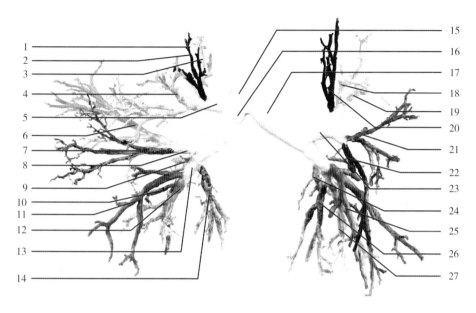

图2-39 肺段支气管（前面观）
pulmonary-segment branches（anterior view）

1. 气管 trachea
2. 肺上叶尖段支气管 apical segmental bronchus
3. 肺上叶后段支气管 posterior segmental bronchus
4. 肺上叶前段支气管 anterior segmental bronchus
5. 右上支气管 right superior segmental bronchus
6. 肺中叶外侧段支气管 lateral segmental bronchus
7. 肺中叶内侧段支气管 medial segmental bronchus
8. 右中叶支气管 right middle lobar bronchus
9. 右肺下叶（尖）上段支气管 right superior segmental bronchus
10. 右肺下叶外侧底段支气管 right lateral segmental bronchus
11. 右肺下叶前底段支气管 right anterior basal segmental bronchus
12. 右肺下叶后底段支气管 right posterior basal segmental bronchus
13. 右下叶支气管 right inferior lobar bronchus
14. 右肺下叶内侧底段支气管 right medial basal segmental bronchus

15. 支气管杈 bifurcation of trachea
16. 右主支气管 right principal bronchus
17. 左主支气管 left principal bronchus
18. 左肺上叶前段支气管 left anterior segmental bronchus
19. 左主支气管 left principal bronchus
20. 左肺上叶尖段支气管 left apical segmental bronchus
21. 左肺上舌段支气管 left superior lingular bronchus
22. 左肺下叶尖支气管 left inferior apical lobar bronchus
23. 左上叶支气管 left superior lobar bronchus
24. 左肺下叶尖上段支气管 left inferior apical suoerior segmental bronchus
25. 左肺下叶前内侧（心底）段支气管 left inferior anterior basal segmental bronchus
26. 左肺下叶后底段支气管 left inferior posterior basal segmental bronchus
27. 左肺下叶外侧底段支气管 left inferior lateral basal segmental bronchus

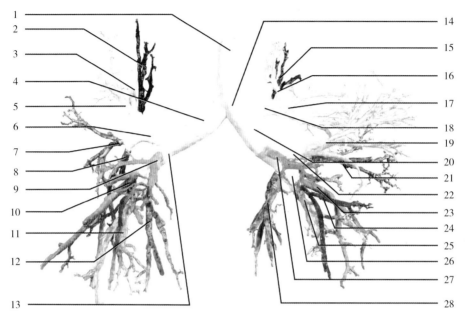

图2-40　肺段支气管（后面观）
pulmonary-segment branches（posterior view）

1. 气管　trachea
2. 尖段支气管　apical segmental bronchus
3. 前段支气管　anterior segmental bronchus
4. 左主支气管　left principal bronchus
5. 后段支气管　posterior segmental bronchus
6. 左上叶支气管　left superior lobar bronchus
7. 上舌段支气管　superior lingular bronchus
8. 下舌段支气管　inferior lingular bronchus
9. 尖上段支气管　apicosuperior segmental bronchus
10. 前内侧（上底）段支气管　anterior basal segmental bronchus
11. 外侧底段支气管　lateral basal segmental bronchus
12. 底段支气管　posterior basal segmental bronchus
13. 左下叶支气管　left inferior lobar bronchus
14. 支气管杈　bifurcation of trachea
15. 尖段支气管　apical segmental bronchus
16. 后段支气管　posterior segmental bronchus
17. 前段支气管　anterior segmental bronchus
18. 右上叶支气管　right superior lobar bronchus
19. 外侧段支气管　lateral segmental bronchus
20. 右主支气管　right principal bronchus
21. 内侧段支气管　medial basal segmental bronchus
22. 右中叶支气管　right middle lobar bronchus
23. 前底段支气管　anterior basal segmental bronchus
24. 外侧底段支气管　lateral basal segmental bronchus
25. 后底段支气管　posterior basal segmental bronchus
26. 右下叶支气管　right inferior lobar bronchus
27. （尖）上段支气管　apicosuperior segmental bronchus
28. 内侧底段支气管　medial basal segmental bronchus

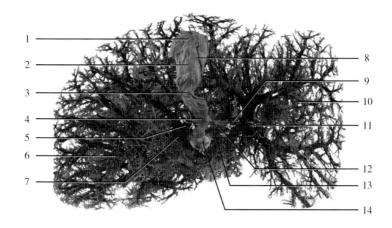

图2-41　肝脏铸型
the cast of liver

1. 胆囊底 fundus of gallbladder
2. 胆囊体 body of gallbladder
3. 胆囊颈 neck of gallbladder
4. 胆囊管 cystic duct
5. 肝右静脉 right hepatic vein
6. 肝右叶 right lobe of liver
7. 右肝管静脉 right trunk of hepatic portal vein

8. 胆囊动脉 cystic artery
9. 肝左动脉 left hepatic artery
10. 肝左叶 left of liver
11. 肝左静脉 left hepatic vein
12. 肝总管 common hepatic duct
13. 左肝管静脉 left trunk of hepatic portal vein
14. 肝门静脉 hepatic portal vein

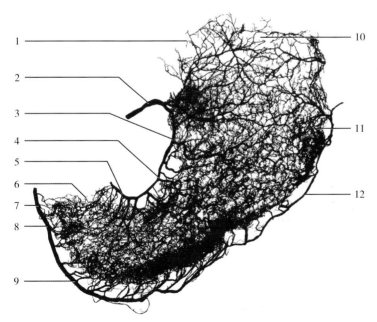

1. 贲门 cardia
2. 胃左动脉 left gastric artery
3. 胃小弯 lesser curvature of stomach
4. 角切迹 angular incisure
5. 胃右动脉 right gastric artery
6. 幽门 pylorus
7. 胃网膜右动脉 right gastroepiploic artery
8. 中间沟 median sulcus
9. 幽门窦 pyloric antrum
10. 胃底 fundus of stomach
11. 胃网膜左动脉 left gastroepiploic artery
12. 胃大弯 greater curvature of stomach

图2-42　胃血管
the blood vessels of stomach

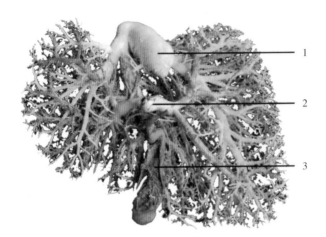

1. 腔静脉 vena cava
2. 门静脉 portal vein
3. 胆囊 gallbladder

图2-43 肝静脉
the hepatic veins

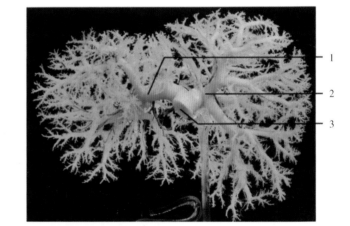

1. 左支 left branch
2. 右支 right branch
3. 门静脉 portal vein

图2-44 门静脉及胆管铸型（下面观）
the cast of hepatic portal vein and bile duct
（inferior view）

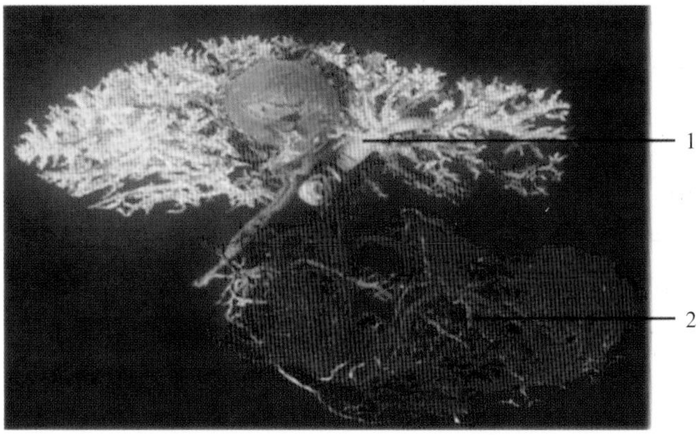

1. 肝门静脉 hepatic portal vein
2. 胃动脉 gastric artery

图2-45 肝门静脉和胃动脉铸型
the cast of hepatic portal vein and gastric artery

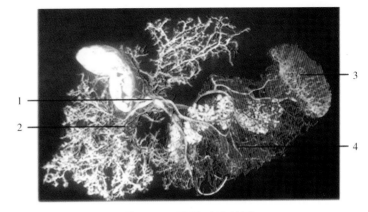

1. 胆管 gallbladder
2. 肝动脉 hepatic artery
3. 脾动脉 splenic artery
4. 胃动脉 gastric artery

图2-46 腹腔动脉铸型
the cast of cleliac artery

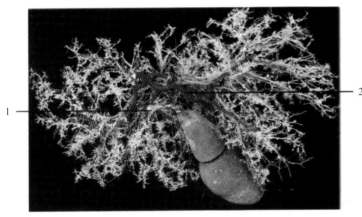

1. 胆管 gallbladder
2. 肝动脉 hepatic artery

图2-47 肝动脉和胆管铸型
the cast of hepatic artery and bile duct

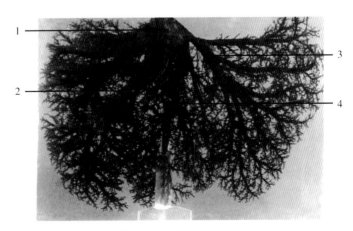

1. 腔静脉 vena cava
2. 肝右静脉 right hepatic vein
3. 肝左静脉 left hepatic vein
4. 肝中静脉 middle hepatic vein

图2-48 肝静脉铸型
the cast of hepatic vein

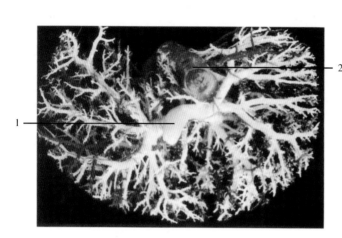

图2-49　肝静脉和门静脉铸型
the cast of hepatic vein and portal vein

1.门静脉　portal vein
2.腔静脉　vena cava

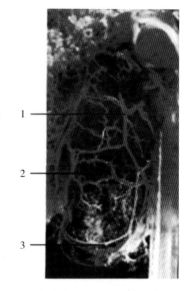

图2-50　胆囊动脉铸型
the cast of gallbladder artery

1.胆囊动脉　cystic artery
2.胆囊　gallbladder
3.胆囊静脉　cystic vein

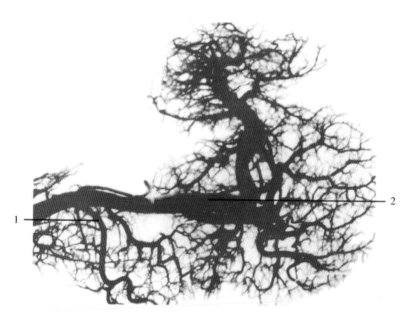

图2-51　脾动脉铸型
the cast of splenic artery

1.胰动脉　pancreas artery　　2.脾动脉　splenic artery

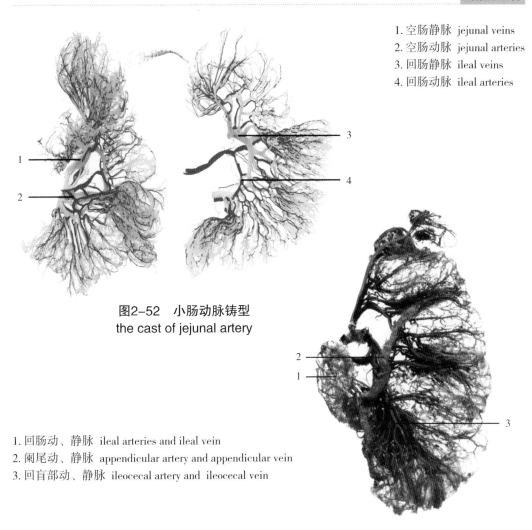

1. 空肠静脉 jejunal veins
2. 空肠动脉 jejunal arteries
3. 回肠静脉 ileal veins
4. 回肠动脉 ileal arteries

图2-52 小肠动脉铸型
the cast of jejunal artery

1. 回肠动、静脉 ileal arteries and ileal vein
2. 阑尾动、静脉 appendicular artery and appendicular vein
3. 回盲部动、静脉 ileocecal artery and ileocecal vein

图2-53 回盲部血管铸型
the cast of ileocecal junction blood vessels

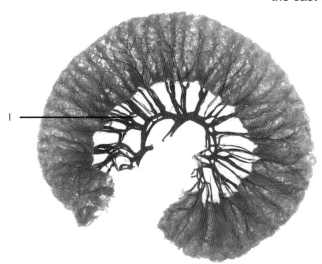

1. 一级动脉弓 primary arteries arch

图2-54 空肠动脉弓（1）
jejunal arteries arch（1）

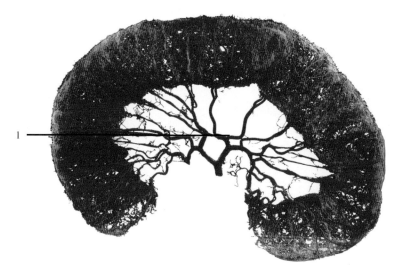

图2-55 空肠动脉弓（2）
jejunal arteries arch（2）

1. 一级动脉弓 primary arteries arch

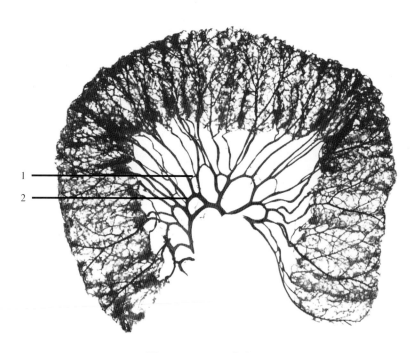

图2-56 回肠动脉弓
ileal arteries arch

1. 二级动脉弓 secondary arteries arch
2. 一级动脉弓 primary arteries arch

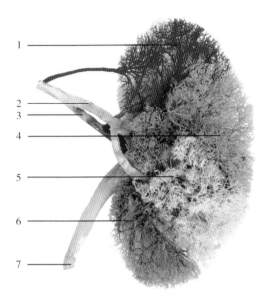

图2-57 肾段动脉分色铸型（前面观）
the dichroic cast of renal–segments
arteries（anterior view）

1. 上段动脉 superior segmental artery
2. 肾动脉前干 anterior renal artery
3. 肾动脉后干 posterior renal artery
4. 上前段动脉 superior anterior segmental artery
5. 下前段动脉 inferior anterior segmental artery
6. 下段动脉 inferior segmental artery
7. 输尿管 ureter

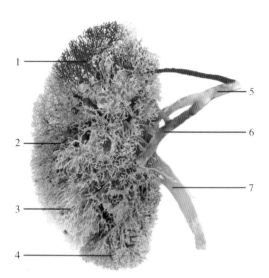

图2-58 肾段动脉分色铸型（后面观）
the dichroic cast of renal–segments
arteries（posterior view）

1. 上段动脉 superior segmental artery
2. 上前段动脉 superior anterior segmental artery
3. 下前段动脉 inferior anterior segmental artery
4. 下段动脉 inferior segmental artery
5. 肾动脉 renal artery
6. 后段动脉 posterior segmental artery
7. 输尿管 ureter

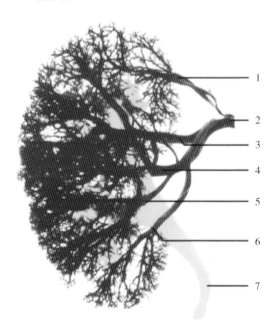

1. 上段动脉 superior segmental artery
2. 肾动脉 renal artery
3. 上前段动脉 superior anterior segmental artery
4. 后支动脉 posterior segmental artery
5. 下前段动脉 inferior anterior segmental artery
6. 下段动脉 inferior segmental artery
7. 输尿管 ureter

图2-59 肾动脉铸型
the cast of renal arteries

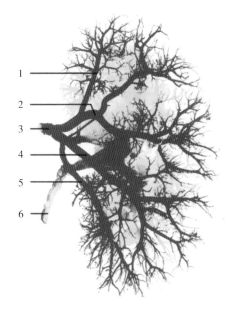

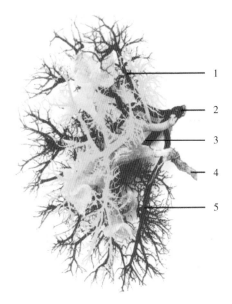

图2-60　肾段动脉铸型（前面观）
the cast of renal–segments arteries
（anterior view）

1. 上段动脉　superior segmental artery
2. 上前段动脉　superior anterior segmental artery
3. 肾动脉　renal artery
4. 下前段动脉　inferior anterior segmental artery
5. 下段动脉　inferior segmental artery
6. 输尿管　ureter

图2-61　肾段动脉铸型（后面观）
the cast of renal–segments arteries
（posterior view）

1. 上段动脉　superior segmental artery
2. 肾动脉　renal artery
3. 后支动脉　posterior segmental artery
4. 输尿管　ureter
5. 下段动脉　inferior segmental artery

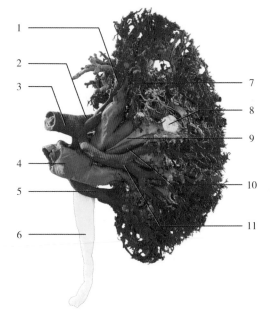

1. 肾上段动脉　renal superior segmental artery
2. 肾后段动脉　renal posterior segmental artery
3. 肾动脉　renal artery
4. 肾静脉　renal vein
5. 肾下段动脉　renal inferior segmental artery
6. 输尿管　ureter
7. 上前段动脉　superior anterior segmental artery
8. 肾小盏　minor renal calices
9. 肾大盏　major renal calices
10. 肾中段动脉　renal medial segmental artery
11. 肾下前段动脉　renal inferior anterior segmental artery

图2-62　肾脏动、静脉铸型（左侧前面观）
the cast of renal arteries and renal veins
（left anterior view）

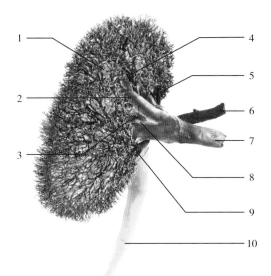

图2-63 肾脏动、静脉铸型（右侧前面观）
the cast of renal arteries and renal veins
（right anterior view）

1. 肾小盏 minor renal calices
2. 肾内静脉 intrarenal vein
3. 下前段动脉 inferior anterior segmental artery
4. 上前段动脉 superior anterior segmental artery
5. 上段动脉 superior segmental artery
6. 肾动脉 renal artery
7. 肾静脉 renal vein
8. 肾盂 renal pelvis
9. 下段动脉 inferior segmental artery
10. 输尿管 ureter

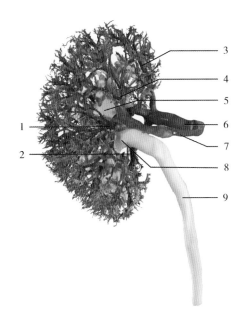

图2-64 肾血管左侧铸型（后面观）
the cast of left renal blood vessels
（posterior view）

1. 肾后段动脉 renal posterior segmental artery
2. 肾下段动脉 renal inferior segmental artery
3. 肾前段动脉 renal anterior segmental artery
4. 肾上前段动脉 renal superior anterior segmental artery
5. 肾大盏 major renal calices
6. 肾动脉 renal artery
7. 肾静脉 renal vein
8. 肾盂 renal pelvis
9. 输尿管动脉 ureter artery

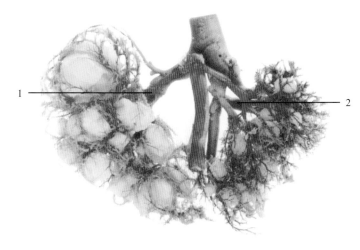

1. 肾动脉 renal artery
2. 肾静脉 renal vein

图2-65 马蹄肾血管铸型（后面观）
the vessels cast of horseshoe kidney （posterior view）

1. 肾动脉 renal artery
2. 肾静脉 renal veins
3. 输尿管 ureter

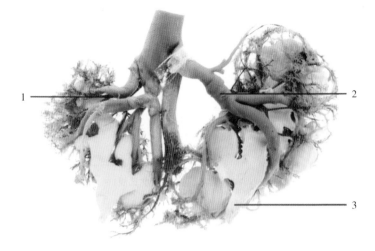

图2-66　马蹄肾血管铸型（前面观）
the vessels cast of horseshoe kidney（anterior view）

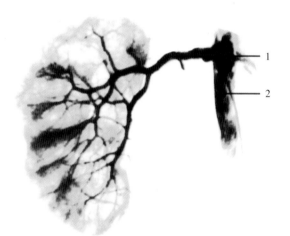

1. 肾动脉 renal artery
2. 腹主动脉 abdominal aorta

图2-67　肾动脉造影
renal artery angiography

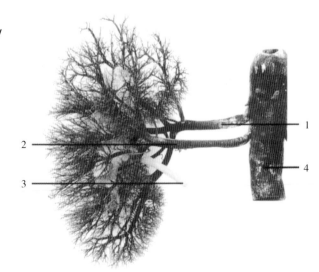

1. 上肾动脉 superior renal artery
2. 下肾动脉 inferior renal artery
3. 输尿管 ureter
4. 腹主动脉 abdominal aorta

图2-68　肾动脉铸型（变异）
the cast of renal arteries（variation）

# 盆部血管

李慧有　林洪春　李洪鹏

吴　敏　吴松林　王　顺

孙国生　甄希成

1. 腹主动脉 abdominal aorta
2. 髂总静脉 common iliac vein
3. 髂内动脉 internal iliac artery
4. 髂外静脉 external iliac vein
5. 髂外动脉 external iliac artery
6. 股动脉 femoral artery
7. 髂总动脉 common iliac artery
8. 髂支 iliac branch
9. 骶外侧静脉
   lateral sacral veins
10. 旋髂深动脉
    deep iliac circumflex artery
11. 股静脉 femoral vein

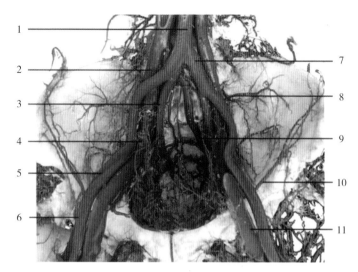

图3-1 骨盆血管铸型
the cast of pelvic vessels

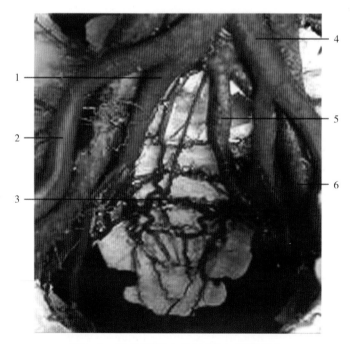

图3-2 骨盆后壁血管铸型（前面观）
the blood vessels cast of pelvic posterior wall（anterior view）

1. 髂内动脉 internal iliac artery    3. 骶静脉丛 sacral venous plexus    5. 骶外侧静脉 lateral sacral veins
2. 髂外动脉 external iliac artery    4. 髂总动脉 common iliac artery    6. 髂外静脉 external iliac vein

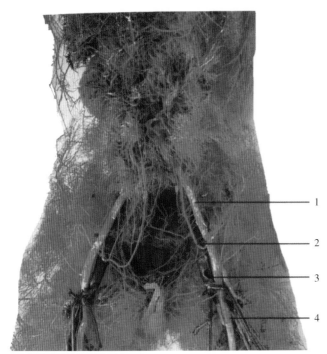

1. 髂外动脉 external iliac artery
2. 腹壁下动脉 inferior epigastric artery
3. 股静脉 femoral vein
4. 股动脉 femoral artery

图3-3　盆部动、静脉铸型
the cast of pelvic arteries and veins

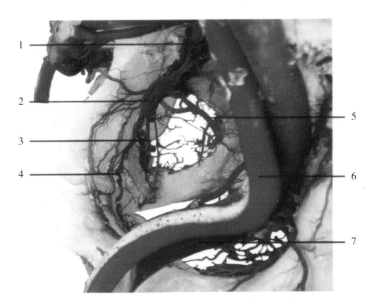

图3-4　闭孔动脉铸型（骨盆内面观1）
the cast of obturator artery（internal view 1）

1. 闭孔动脉 obturator artery
2. 耻骨支 pubic branch
3. 闭孔动脉前支 anterior branch of obturator artery
4. 耻骨静脉丛 pubic venous plexus
5. 闭孔动脉后支 posterior branch of obturator artery
6. 髂外动脉 external iliac artery
7. 髂外静脉 external iliac vein

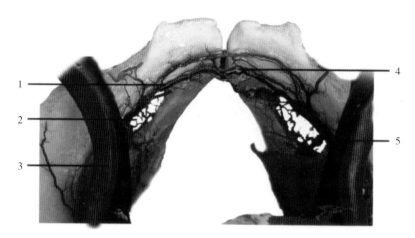

**图3-5 闭孔动脉铸型（骨盆内面观2）**
the cast of obturator artery（internal view 2）

1. 耻骨支（闭孔动脉） pubic branch　　4. 耻骨后静脉丛 retropubic venous
2. 闭孔 obturator foramen　　　　　　5. 髂外静脉 external iliac vein
3. 髂外动脉 external iliac artery

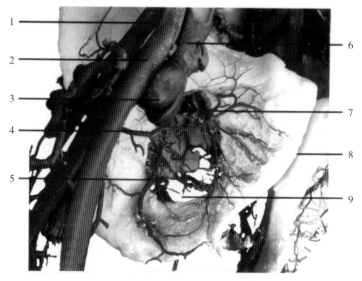

**图3-6 闭孔动脉铸型（外面观）**
the cast of obturator artery（external view）

1. 股深动脉 deep femoral artery　　　　6. 股静脉 femoral vein
2. 股动脉 femoral artery　　　　　　　7. 闭孔动脉前支 anterior branch of obturator artery
3. 静脉瓣 venous valve　　　　　　　　8. 耻骨联合 pubic symphysis
4. 旋股内侧动脉 medial femoral circumflex artery　9. 闭孔 obturator foramen
5. 闭孔动脉后支 posterior branch of obturator artery

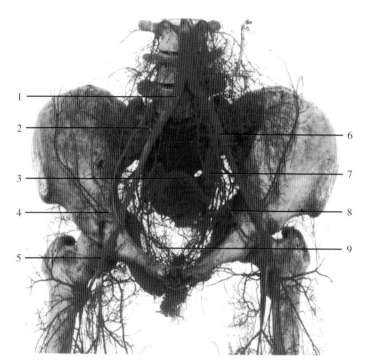

1. 髂总动脉 common iliac artery
2. 髂腰动脉 iliolumbar artery
3. 子宫动脉丛 uterine artery rete
4. 旋髂深动脉
   deep iliac circumflex artery
5. 股动脉 femoral artery
6. 髂外动脉 external iliac artery
7. 卵巢动脉 ovarian artery
8. 腹壁下动脉 inferior epigastric
   artery
9. 膀胱动脉丛 bladder artery
   rete

图3-7 女性盆部动脉铸型（前面观1）
the cast of female pelvic arteries（anterior view 1）

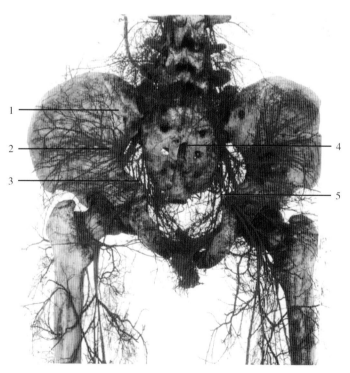

1. 髂骨 ilium
2. 臀上动脉 superior gluteal
   artery
3. 臀下动脉 inferior gluteal artery
4. 骶骨 sacrum
5. 阴部内动脉 internal pudendal
   artery

图3-8 女性盆部动脉铸型（后面观）
the cast of female pelvic arteries（posterior view）

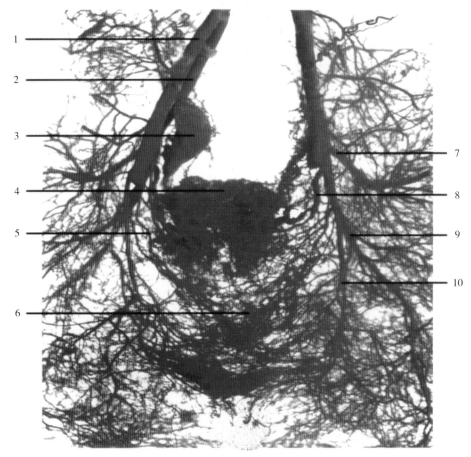

**图3-9　女性盆部动脉铸型（前面观2）**
the cast of female pelvic arteries（anterior view 2）

1. 髂外动脉　external iliac artery
2. 髂内动脉　internal iliac artery
3. 卵巢动脉　ovarian artery
4. 子宫动脉丛　uterine artery rete
5. 膀胱动脉　bladder artery
6. 膀胱动脉丛　bladder artery rete
7. 臀上动脉　superior gluteal artery
8. 子宫动脉　uterine artery
9. 臀下动脉　inferior gluteal artery
10. 阴部内动脉　internal pudendal artery

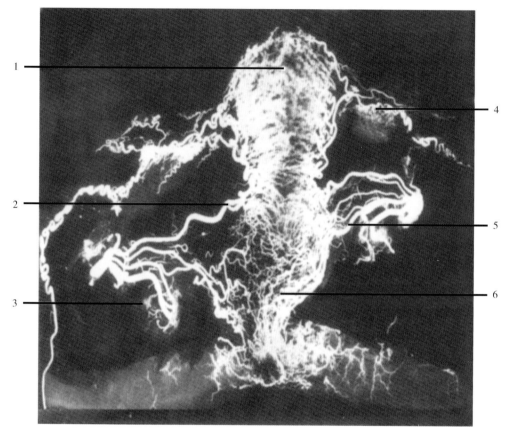

图3-10　子宫动脉造影
uterine artery angiography

1. 子宫动脉丛　uterine artery rete
2. 子宫动脉　uterine artery
3. 卵巢动脉　ovarian artery
4. 卵巢动脉丛　ovarian artery rete
5. 阴道动脉　vaginal artery
6. 阴道动脉丛　vaginal artery rete

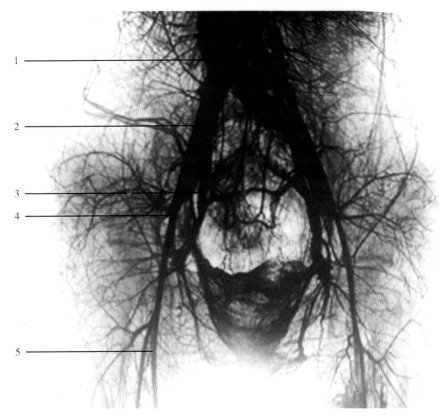

图3-11　女性盆部动脉造影
female pelvic arteries angiography

1.腹主动脉 abdominal aorta
2.髂总动脉 common iliac artery
3.髂内动脉 internal iliac artery
4.髂外动脉 external iliac artery
5.股动脉 femoral artery

# 上肢血管

高　岩　孙永林　郭中献
孙翔宇　甄希成　陈　新
孙国生　郑　岩

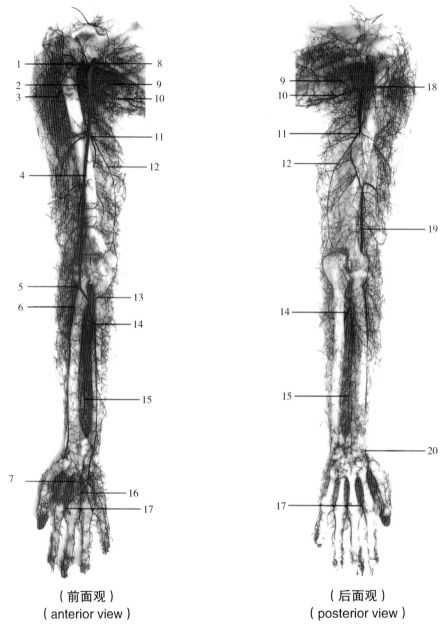

（前面观）
（anterior view）

（后面观）
（posterior view）

图4-1　上肢动脉铸型
the cast of upper limb arteries

1. 胸肩峰动脉　thoracoacromial artery
2. 旋肱前动脉　anterior humeral circumflex artery
3. 旋肱后动脉　posterior humeral circumflex artery
4. 肱动脉　brachial artery
5. 桡侧返动脉　radial recurrent artery
6. 桡动脉　radial artery
7. 掌深弓　deep palmar arch
8. 腋动脉　axillary artery
9. 旋肩胛动脉　circumflex scapular artery
10. 胸背动脉　thoracodorsal artery

11. 肱深动脉　deep brachial artery
12. 尺侧上副动脉　superior ulnar collateral artery
13. 尺侧返动脉　ulnar recurrent artery
14. 尺动脉　ulnar artery
15. 骨间背侧动脉　lateral interosseous artery
16. 掌浅弓　superficial palmar arch
17. 指掌侧总动脉　common palmar digital arteries
18. 旋肱后动脉　posterior humeral circumflex artery
19. 肱动脉　brachial artery
20. 桡动脉　radial artery

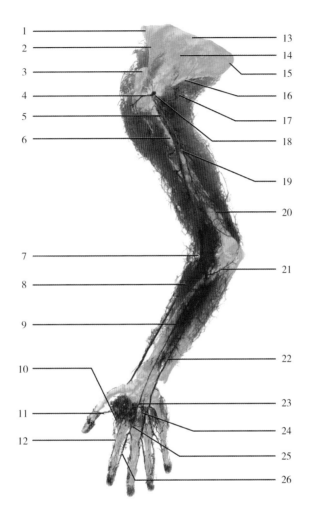

图4-2 上肢血管铸型
the cast of upper limb vessels

1. 肩胛骨上角 superior angle of scapula
2. 上缘 superior border
3. 喙突 coracoid process
4. 肩峰 thoracoacromion
5. 旋肱前动脉 anterior humeral circumflex artery
6. 肱动脉 brachial artery
7. 桡侧返动脉 radial recurrent artery
8. 桡动脉 radial artery
9. 骨间前动脉 anterior interosseous artery
10. 指掌侧总动脉 common palmar digital arteries
11. 拇主要动脉 principal artery of thumb
12. 示指桡侧动脉 radial artery of index
13. 内侧缘 medial border

14. 肩胛下窝 subscapular fossa
15. 肩胛骨下角 inferior angle of scapula
16. 外侧缘 lateral border
17. 腋动脉 axillary artery
18. 肩胛下动脉 subscapular artery
19. 尺侧上副动脉 superior ulnar collateral artery
20. 尺侧下副动脉 inferior ulnar collateral artery
21. 尺侧返动脉 ulnar recurrent artery
22. 尺动脉 ulnar artery
23. 掌深弓 deep palmar arch
24. 掌浅弓 superficial palmar arch
25. 指掌侧总动脉 common palmar digital artery
26. 指间动脉 interfingual artery

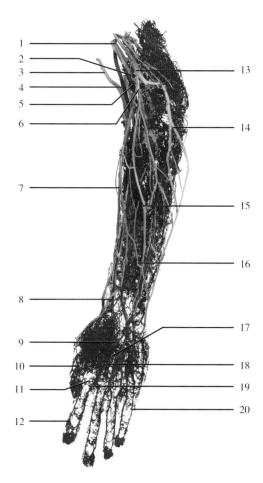

1. 桡静脉 radial vein
2. 尺静脉 ulnar vein
3. 头静脉 cephalic vein
4. 桡动脉 radial artery
5. 尺动脉 ulnar artery
6. 肘正中静脉 median cubital vein
7. 头静脉 cephalic vein
8. 桡动脉 radial artery
9. 拇主要动脉 principal artery of thumb
10. 拇指桡侧动脉 radial artery of thumb
11. 拇指尺掌侧动脉 ulnar palmar thumb collateral artery
12. 示指桡侧动脉 radial artery of index
13. 贵要静脉 basilic vein
14. 头静脉 cephalic vein
15. 前臂正中静脉 median antebrachial vein
16. 尺静脉 ulnar vein
17. 掌深弓 deep palmar arch
18. 掌浅弓 superficial palmar arch
19. 掌心动脉 palmar metacarpal arteries
20. 小指尺掌侧动脉 ulnar digital minimi artery

图4-3 上肢动、静脉铸型
the cast of upper limb arteries and veins

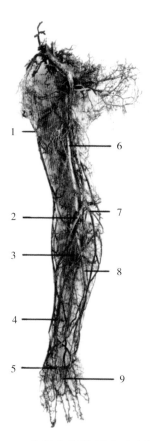

图4-4 上肢血管铸型（酸腐蚀）
the cast of upper limb vessels
（acid corrosion）

1. 头静脉 cephalic vein
2. 肘正中静脉 median cubital vein
3. 前臂正中静脉 median antebrachial vein
4. 桡动脉 radial artery
5. 掌深弓 deep palmar arch
6. 肱动脉 brachial artery
7. 贵要静脉 basilic vein
8. 尺动脉 ulnar artery
9. 掌浅弓 superficial palmar arch

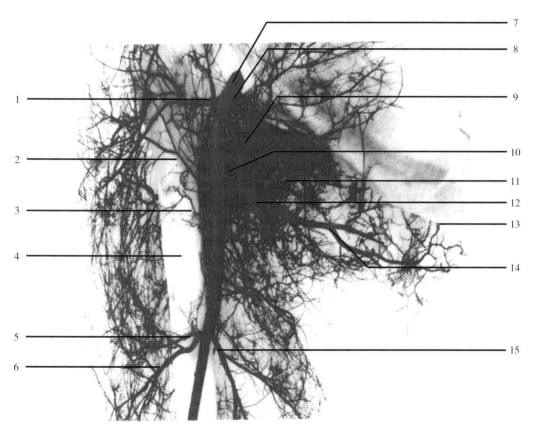

图4-5　肩部血管铸型
the cast of shoulder vessels

1. 胸肩峰动脉 thoracoacromial artery
2. 旋肱前动脉 anterior humeral circumflex artery
3. 肱深动脉 deep brachial artery
4. 肱骨 the humerus
5. 肱骨滋养动脉 humeral nutrient arteries
6. 桡侧上副动脉 superior radial collateral artery
7. 腋动脉 axillary artery
8. 胸上动脉 superior thoracic artery

9. 胸外侧动脉 lateral thoracic artery
10. 旋肱后动脉 posterior humeral circumflex artery
11. 旋肩胛动脉 circumflex scapular artery
12. 肩胛下动脉 subscapular artery
13. 肩胛下角 inferior angle of scapula
14. 胸前动脉 anterior thoracic artery
15. 尺侧上副动脉 superior ulnar collateral artery

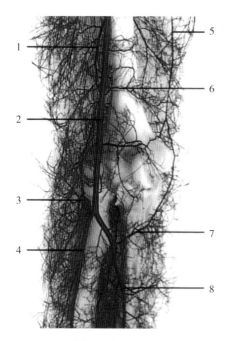

1. 桡侧上副动脉 superior radial collateral artery
2. 肱动脉 brachial artery
3. 桡侧返动脉 radial recurrent artery
4. 桡动脉 radial artery
5. 尺侧上副动脉 superior ulnar collateral artery
6. 尺侧下副动脉 inferior ulnar collateral artery
7. 尺侧返动脉 ulnar recurrent artery
8. 尺动脉 ulnar artery

图4-6　肘部动脉铸型（前面观）
the cast of arteries of cubital portion（anterior view）

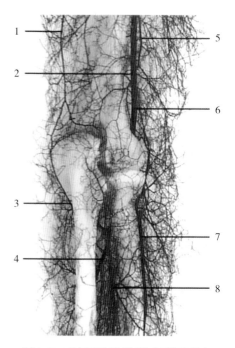

1. 尺侧上副动脉 superior ulnar collateral artery
2. 尺侧下副动脉 inferior ulnar collateral artery
3. 尺侧返动脉 ulnar recurrent artery
4. 尺动脉 ulnar artery
5. 桡侧下副动脉 inferior radial collateral artery
6. 肱动脉 brachial artery
7. 桡动脉 radial artery
8. 骨间总动脉 common interosseous artery

图4-7　肘部动脉铸型（后面观）
the cast of arteries of cubital portion
（posterior view）

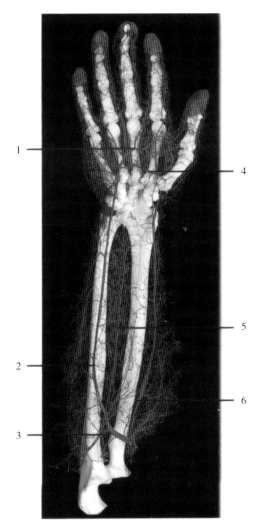

图4-8　前臂动脉铸型（自然腐蚀）
the cast of forearm arteries（natural corrosion）

1. 掌浅弓　superficial palmar arch
2. 尺动脉　ulnar artery
3. 尺侧返动脉　ulnar recurrent artery
4. 掌深弓　deep palmar arch
5. 骨间前动脉　anterior interosseous artery
6. 桡动脉　radial artery

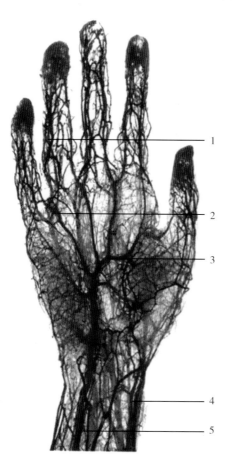

1. 指掌侧固有动脉 proper palmar digital arteries
2. 指掌侧总动脉 common palmar digital arteries
3. 掌浅弓 superficial palmar arch
4. 桡动脉 radial artery
5. 尺动脉 ulnar artery

图4-9 手部血管铸型（前面观）
the cast of blood vessels in hand
（anterior view）

1. 指背静脉网 dorsal digital venous rete
2. 手背静脉网 dorsal venous rete of hand

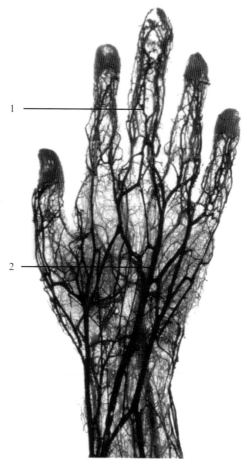

图4-10 手部血管铸型（后面观）
the cast of blood vessels in hand
（posterior view）

1. 指掌侧总动脉 common palmar digital arteries
2. 掌浅弓 superficial palmar arch
3. 掌浅支 superficial palmar branch
4. 尺动脉 ulnar artery
5. 掌心动脉 palmar metacarpal arteries
6. 掌深弓 deep palmar arch
7. 掌浅支 superficial palmar branch
8. 桡动脉 radial artery

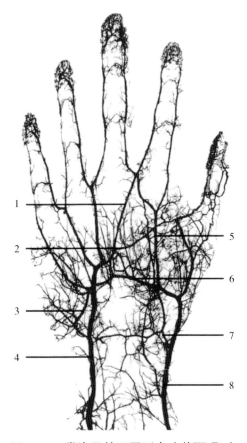

图4-11　掌浅弓的不同形态（前面观1）
different forms of superficial palmar arch
（anterior view 1）

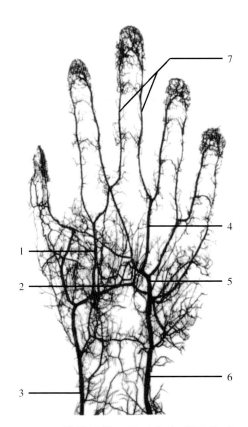

图4-12　掌浅弓的不同形态（后面观1）
different forms of superficial palmar arch
（posterior view 1）

1. 掌心动脉 palmar metacarpal arteries
2. 掌深弓 deep palmar arch
3. 桡动脉 radial artery
4. 掌浅弓 superficial palmar arch
5. 指掌侧总动脉 common palmar digital arteries
6. 尺动脉 ulnar artery
7. 指掌侧固有动脉 proper palmar digital arteries

1. 掌心动脉 palmar metacarpal arteries
2. 掌浅弓 superficial palmar arch
3. 掌深支 deep palmar branch
4. 桡动脉 radial artery
5. 指掌侧总动脉 common palmar digital arteries
6. 掌深弓 deep palmar arch
7. 尺动脉 ulnar artery

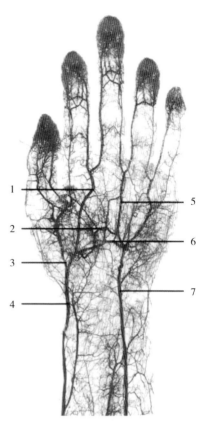

图4-13 掌浅弓的不同形态（前面观2）
different forms of superficial palmar arch
（anterior view 2）

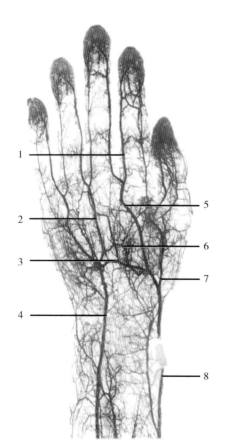

图4-14 掌浅弓的不同形态（后面观2）
different forms of superficial palmar arch
（posterior view 2）

1. 指掌侧固有动脉 proper palmar digital arteries
2. 指掌侧总动脉 common palmar digital arteries
3. 掌深弓 deep palmar arch
4. 尺动脉 ulnar artery
5. 掌心动脉 palmar metacarpal arteries
6. 掌浅弓 superficial palmar arch
7. 掌深支 deep palmar branch
8. 桡动脉 radial artery

1. 掌浅弓 superficial palmar arch
2. 掌深支 deep palmar branch
3. 尺动脉 ulnar artery
4. 指掌侧总动脉 common palmar digital arteries
5. 掌心动脉 palmar metacarpal arteries
6. 掌浅支 superficial palmar branch
7. 掌深弓 deep palmar arch
8. 桡动脉 radial artery

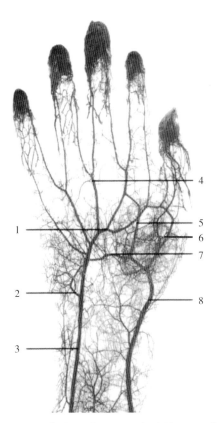

图4-15 掌浅弓的不同形态（前面观3）
different forms of superficial palmar arch
（ anterior view 3 ）

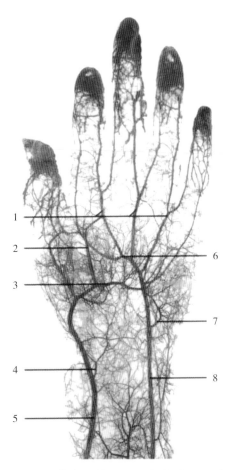

1. 指掌侧总动脉 common palmar digital arteries
2. 掌心动脉 palmar metacarpal arteries
3. 掌深弓 deep palmar arch
4. 掌浅支 superficial palmar branch
5. 桡动脉 radial artery
6. 掌浅弓 superficial palmar arch
7. 掌深支 deep palmar branch
8. 尺动脉 ulnar artery

图4-16 掌浅弓的不同形态（后面观3）
different forms of superficial palmar arch
（ posterior view 3 ）

1. 指掌侧固有动脉 proper palmar digital arteries
2. 指掌侧总动脉 common palmar digital arteries
3. 掌浅弓 superficial palmar arch
4. 正中动脉 median artery
5. 尺动脉 ulnar artery
6. 掌心动脉 palmar metacarpal arteries
7. 掌深弓 deep palmar arch
8. 掌浅支 superficial palmar branch
9. 桡动脉 radial artery

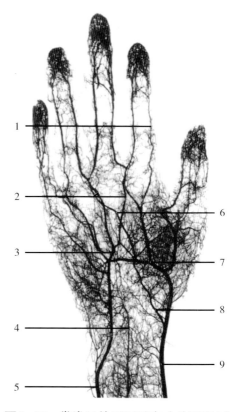

图4-17 掌浅弓的不同形态（前面观4）
different forms of superficial palmar arch
（anterior view 4）

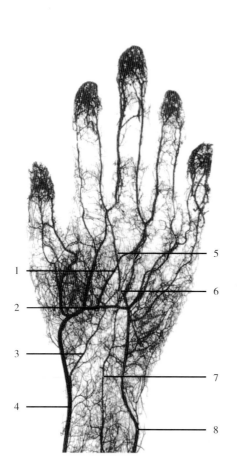

图4-18 掌浅弓的不同形态（后面观4）
different forms of superficial palmar arch
（posterior view 4）

1. 掌心动脉 palmar metacarpal arteries
2. 掌深弓浅弓 superficial arch of deep palmar arch
3. 掌浅弓深弓 superficial palmar arch
4. 桡动脉 radial artery
5. 指掌侧总动脉 common palmar digital arteries
6. 掌浅弓 superficial palmar arch
7. 正中动脉 median artery
8. 尺动脉 ulnar artery

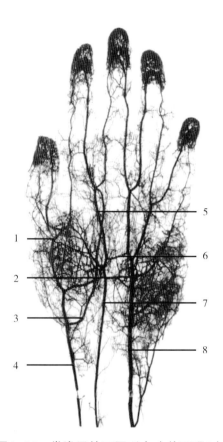

1. 拇主要动脉 principal artery of thumb
2. 掌深弓 deep palmar arch
3. 掌背动脉 dorsal metacarpal artery
4. 桡动脉 radial artery
5. 指掌侧总动脉 common palmar digital arteries
6. 掌浅弓 superficial palmar arch
7. 正中动脉 median artery
8. 尺动脉 ulnar artery

图4-19　掌浅弓的不同形态（前面观5）
different forms of superficial palmar arch
（anterior view 5）

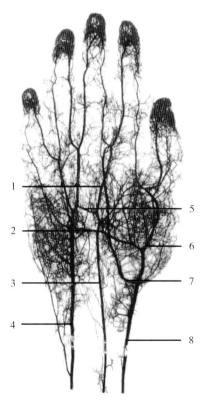

1. 指掌侧总动脉 common palmar digital arteries
2. 掌深弓 deep palmar arch
3. 正中动脉 median artery
4. 尺动脉 ulnar artery
5. 掌浅弓 superficial palmar arch
6. 拇主要动脉 principal artery of thumb
7. 掌背动脉 dorsal metacarpal arteriy
8. 桡动脉 radial artery

图4-20　掌浅弓的不同形态（后面观5）
different forms of superficial palmar arch
（posterior view 5）

1. 掌心动脉 palmar metacarpal arteries
2. 掌浅弓 superficial palmar arch
3. 掌浅支 superficial palmar branch
4. 桡动脉终支 terminal branch of radial artery
5. 桡动脉 radial artery
6. 指掌侧总动脉 common palmar digital arteries
7. 掌深弓 deep palmar arch
8. 掌深支 deep palmar branch
9. 尺动脉 ulnar artery

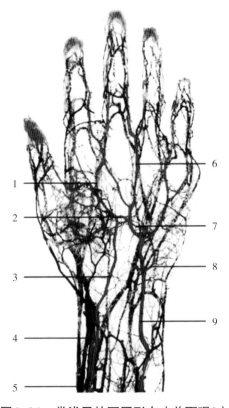

图4-21　掌浅弓的不同形态（前面观6）
different forms of superficial palmar arch
（anterior view 6）

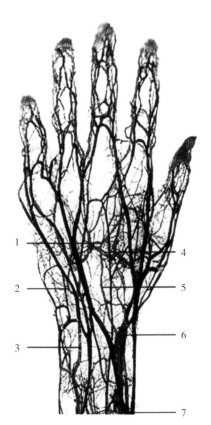

图4-22　掌浅弓的不同形态（后面观6）
different forms of superficial palmar arch
（posterior view 6）

1. 掌浅弓 superficial palmar arch
2. 掌深支 deep palmar branch
3. 尺动脉 ulnar artery
4. 掌深弓 deep palmar arch
5. 掌浅支 superficial palmar branch
6. 桡动脉终支 terminal branch of radial artery
7. 桡动脉 radial artery

1. 指掌侧总动脉 common palmar digital arteries
2. 掌浅弓 superficial palmar arch
3. 尺动脉 ulnar artery
4. 桡动脉 radial artery

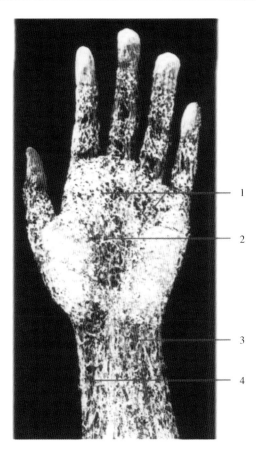

图4-23 掌浅弓的不同形态皮下浅层（前面观）
different forms of superficial palmar arch
（anterior view）

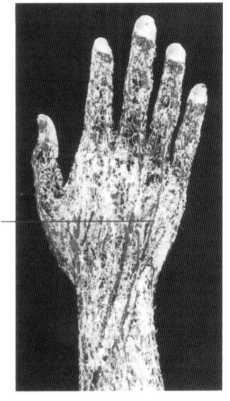

1. 掌背静脉网 dorsal metacarpal venous rete

图4-24 掌浅弓的不同形态皮下浅层（后面观）
different forms of superficial palmar arch
（posterior view）

1. 掌浅弓 superficial palmar arch
2. 掌深弓 deep palmar arch
3. 尺动脉 ulnar artery
4. 拇主要动脉 principal artery of thumb
5. 桡动脉 radial artery
6. 正中动脉 median artery

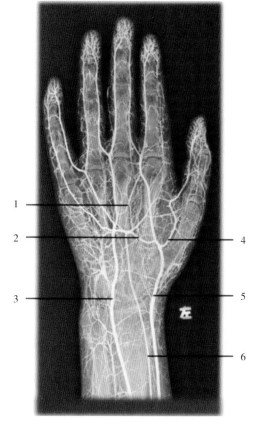

图4-25 掌浅弓的不同形态造影（后面观1）
different forms of superficial palmar arch
（posterior view 1）

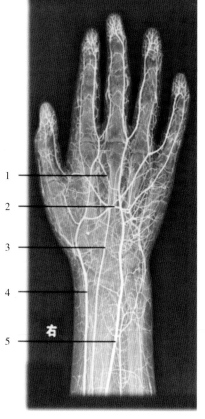

图4-26 掌浅弓的不同形态造影（后面观2）
different forms of superficial palmar arch
（posterior view 2）

1. 掌浅弓 superficial palmar arch
2. 掌深弓 deep palmar arch
3. 正中动脉 median artery
4. 桡动脉 radial artery
5. 尺动脉 ulnar artery

# 下肢血管

孙国生　吴松林　高　岩
吴　敏　佟　瑶　陈　新
郑　岩　甄希成

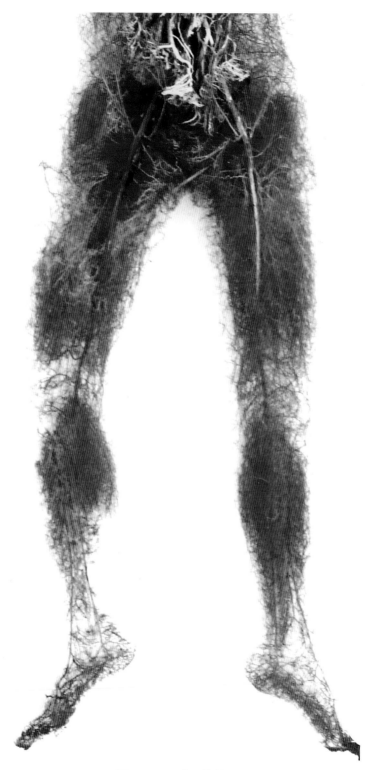

图5-1　下肢血管铸型
the cast of lower limb blood vessels

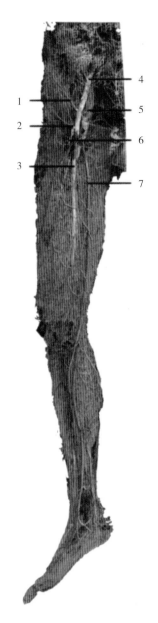

**图5-2　下肢血管铸型（酸腐蚀）**
the cast of lower limb blood vessels
（acid corrosion）

1. 旋髂深动脉 deep iliac circumflex artery
2. 旋髂浅动脉 superficial iliac circumflex artery
3. 股动脉 femoral artery
4. 髂外动脉 external iliac artery
5. 腹壁下动脉 inferior epigastric artery
6. 股深动脉 deep femoral artery
7. 大隐静脉 great saphenous vein

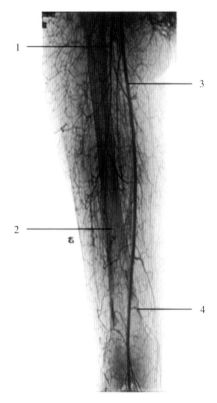

**图5-3　股部动脉造影**
angiography of femoral arteries

1. 股深动脉 deep femoral artery
2. 股骨 femur
3. 股动脉 femoral artery
4. 膝降动脉 descending genicular artery

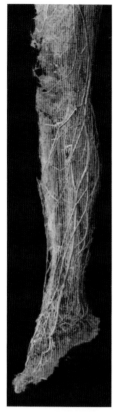

图5-4 腿血管铸型（酸腐蚀）
the cast of leg vessels
（acid corrosion）

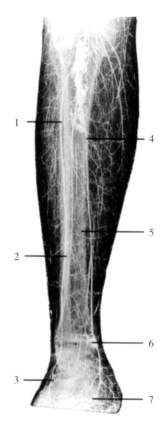

图5-5 小腿动脉造影
leg artery angiography

1. 胫前动脉 anterior tibial artery
2. 腓骨 fibula
3. 足背动脉 dorsal artery of foot
4. 胫后动脉 posterior tibial artery
5. 胫骨 tibia
6. 内踝 medial malleolus
7. 足底动脉 plantar artery

1. 跗内侧动脉 medial tarsal artery
2. 足底内侧动脉 medial plantar artery
3. 胫后动脉 posterior tibial artery
4. 跟骨支 calcaneal branch
5. 足底外侧动脉 lateral plantar artery

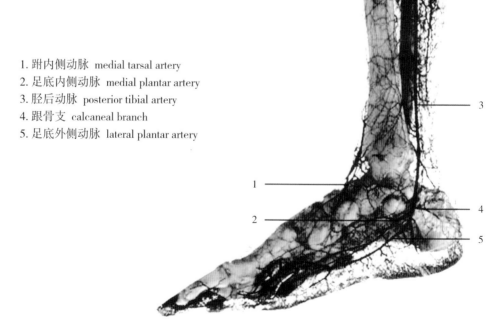

图5-6 足部动脉铸型（自然腐蚀）
the cast of foot arteries（natural corrosion）

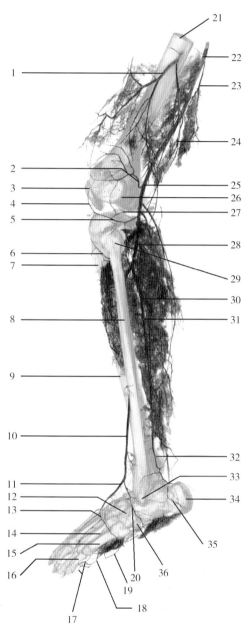

图5-7　下肢血管铸型
the cast of lower limb arteries

1. 旋股外侧动脉　lateral femoral circumflex artery
2. 膝上外侧动脉　lateral superior genicular artery
3. 髌骨　patella
4. 髌动脉网　patellar artery rete
5. 膝下外侧动脉　lateral inferior genicular artery
6. 胫前返动脉　anterior tibial recurrent artery
7. 胫骨粗隆　tuberosity of tibia
8. 腓骨　fibula
9. 胫骨　tibia
10. 胫前动脉　anterior tibial artery
11. 足背动脉　dorsal artery of foot
12. 楔骨　cuneiform bone
13. 弓状动脉　arcuate artery
14. 跖背动脉　dorsal metatarsal arteries
15. 跖骨　metatarsal bone
16. 趾骨　phalanx
17. 趾足底固有动脉　proper plantar digital artery
18. 跖足底总动脉　common plantar digital artery
19. 足底外侧动脉　lateral plantar artery
20. 跗外侧动脉　lateral tarsal artery
21. 股骨　femur
22. 股动脉　femoral artery
23、24. 穿动脉　perforating arteries
25. 腘动脉　popliteal artery
26. 外侧髁　lateral condyle
27. 髁间隆起　mtercondylar eminence
28. 胫后动脉　posterior tibial artery
29. 腓骨头　fibular head
30. 胫后动脉　posterior tibial artery
31. 腓动脉　peroneal artery
32. 腓动脉穿支　peroneal perforating branch artery
33. 外踝　lateral malleolus
34. 跟骨　calcaneus
35. 跟动脉网　calcaneal artery rete
36. 骰骨　cuboid bone

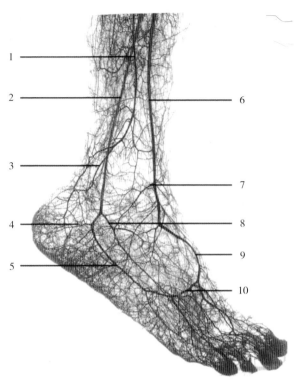

1. 腓动脉 peroneal artery
2. 胫后动脉 posterior tibial artery
3. 外踝支 lateral malleolar branches
4. 跟网 calcaneal rete
5. 足底外侧动脉 lateral plantar artery
6. 胫前动脉 anterior tibial artery
7. 跗外侧动脉 lateral tarsal artery
8. 足底内侧动脉 medial plantar artery
9. 足背动脉 dorsal artery of foot
10. 足底弓 plantar arch

图5-8　足部动脉铸型（外面观，酸腐蚀）
the cast of foot arteries（external view and acid corrosion）

1. 腓动脉 peroneal artery
2. 胫前动脉 anterior tibial artery
3. 跗外侧动脉 lateral tarsal artery
4. 足底内侧动脉 medial plantar artery
5. 足背动脉 dorsal artery of foot
6. 足底弓 plantar arch
7. 胫后动脉 posterior tibial artery
8. 外踝支 lateral malleolar branches
9. 跟骨支 calcaneal branch
10. 足底外侧动脉 lateral plantar artery

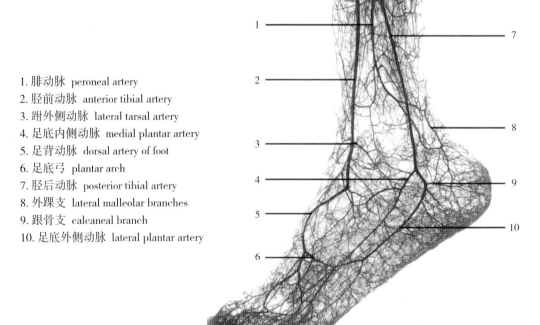

图5-9　足部动脉铸型（内面观，酸腐蚀）
the cast of foot arteries（internal view and acid corrosion）

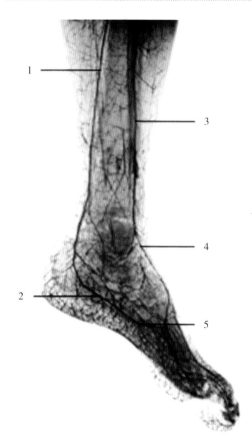

1. 胫后动脉 posterior tibial artery
2. 足底动脉 plantar artery
3. 胫前动脉 anterior tibial artery
4. 足背动脉 dorsal artery of foot
5. 足底弓 plantar arch

图5-10　足部动脉造影（1）
foot arteries angiography（1）

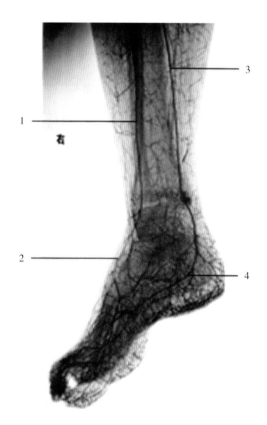

1. 胫前动脉 anterior tibial artery
2. 足背动脉 dorsal artery of foot
3. 胫后动脉 posterior tibial artery
4. 足底动脉 plantar artery

图5-11　足部动脉造影（2）
foot arteries angiography（2）

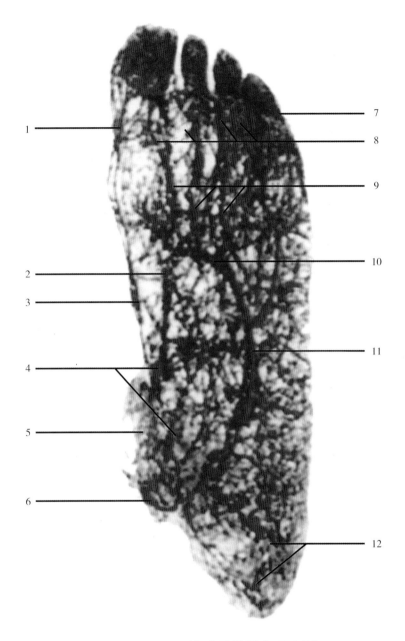

### 图5-12 足部血管铸型（下面观）
the cast foot blood vessels（inferior view）

1. 跗趾固有动脉 proper hallucis artery
2. 深支 deep branch
3. 浅支 superficial branch
4. 足底内侧动脉 medial plantar artery
5. 内踝网 medial malleolar rete
6. 胫后动脉 posterior tibial artery

7. 小趾固有动脉 proper digiti minimi artery
8. 趾足底固有动脉 proper plantar digital artery
9. 趾足底总动脉 common plantar digital artery
10. 足底动静脉弓 plantar artery arch and vein arch
11. 足底外侧动静脉 lateral plantar artery and vein
12. 动、静脉跟网 calcaneal artery and vein rete